Women *and* Health

· *in* ·

AFRICA

Edited by

Meredeth Turshen

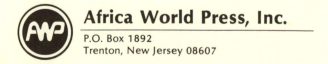

Africa World Press, Inc.

P.O. Box 1892
Trenton, New Jersey 08607

Africa World Press, Inc.

P.O. Box 1892
Trenton, New Jersey 08607

Copyright © 1991 Meredeth Turshen
First Printing 1991

Book design and typesetting by Malcolm Litchfield
This book is composed in Sabon

Cover design by Charles Juzang
Cover photo courtesy of the United Nations

Library of Congress Catalog Card Number: 90-81573

ISBN: 0-86543-180-9   Cloth
         0-86543-181-7   Paper

Contents

Acknowledgments

THE LOGISTICS of putting this book together were especially difficult because the authors were scattered across three continents. I sometimes suspected the international postal services of sabotaging our work. There was political interference—research materials were confiscated by the police; and there were domestic casualties—divorce prevented two manuscripts from being completed. Working with African women and putting their views across as clearly as possible were important to me. I am very grateful to all of the contributors who responded so positively to my editorial intrusions.

My sense of relief in finishing this book brings out strong feelings of gratitude towards everyone who helped, directly or indirectly, in its production. Thanks to the Department of Urban Studies at Rutgers University, I was able to spend this year abroad, working on this book and other projects. Thanks to a grant from the Rutgers University Reseach Council, I was able to travel to Paris, where this work was completed.

L'Institut National de la Santé et de la Recherche Médicale (INSERM) was my host for the year, and I am grateful to l'Unité 292 (Public Health, Epidemiology, and Human Reproduction), which provided essential research and writing facilities. My deepest thanks go to Annie Thébaud-Mony who invited me to work with her at INSERM this year, and to the équipe ISIS (Inégalités sociales, industrialisation, et santé), whose warm welcome made these months interesting and enjoyable. Merci!

A number of people helped by reading drafts, suggesting contacts, and supplying references: grateful thanks to Hélène Bretin, Pierre and Claudine Chaulet, Lamine Cissé, Christian Clanet, Sally Cornwell, Michel François, Thérèse Locoh, Shula Marks, Erika Royston, and Annie Thébaud-Mony. Thanks also to the members of two reading groups—ISIS Femmes and MF IV—who will find the themes of many discussions reflected in these pages.

A year away is not possible without the support of family, friends, and colleagues. I am grateful to you all, and especially to Cecile Shore and Tony Astrachan.

Meredeth Turshen
Paris, July 14, 1990

· 1 ·

Introduction

MEREDETH TURSHEN

THIS IS A BOOK about the multiplicity of health problems that African women experience as a result of the many ways in which they contribute to African society and as a direct consequence of the impact of large political and economic forces on their lives. The primary focus is the broad issues that affect women's health—war and revolution, the economy and work, population growth and demographic controls, health services and disease control programs. The authors emphasize the general problems of the communities in which women live, work, marry, divorce, and bear and raise children.

Many chapters are based on fieldwork; nonetheless, the analysis is pitched at the macrosocial level in order to portray women accurately in the place they occupy in African affairs. Each specific health issue—nutrition, AIDS, occupational disease, birth control—is discussed in a country context. The concluding chapter addresses the issues of health services in a general framework. Many of the authors are African and most let African women speak for themselves; details from the lives of individual women personalize several contributions. All of the studies concern African women as active participants in their political economies, their struggles for empowerment, and the obstacles they encounter in their quest for better lives for themselves and their children. The solutions proposed embrace public health and development programs, as distinct from individual medical care.

The book samples most parts of Africa, although geographical representation is not a primary concern. The case studies report on women in Algeria, Côte d'Ivoire, Mozambique, Namibia, Nigeria, South Africa, Zaire, and Zimbabwe. The concluding chapter draws upon the experiences of women in Burkina Faso, Mali, Mauritania, Niger, Senegal, and Western Sahara. This diversified selection of countries overcomes a tendency to present regional studies from only one of the former European empires, which perpetuates the colonial divisions of Africa.

Approaches to Women's Health

Broadly speaking, there appear to be two major streams of thought in contemporary feminist theory: one emphasizes the psychological development of women and the other the material conditions that determine gender differentiation. Writers such as Jessica Benjamin, Nancy Chodorow, Carol Gilligan, Luce Irigary, Juliette Mitchell, and Christiane Olivier represent the first tendency. They hold that women are subordinate to men because of the different early maternal experiences of male and female infants, and because mothering is conditioned by patriarchy and sexist social attitudes. Those psychological theorists influenced by Freud add to infantile experiences the Oedipal/Electra complex of family dynamics in early childhood, which conditions women to be submissive and trains men to dominate. The authors usually acknowledge the ethnocentricity of their studies and question the applicability or relevance of their findings to societies that do not place a high value on individualism. Some third world feminists such as Fatima

Mernissi use these tools to analyze their societies, but others, following Frantz Fanon, find psychoanalytic theory unable to explain the dynamics of subordination in colonized societies.

Leith Mullings, Sheila Rowbotham, Karen Sacks, and Kate Young represent the materialist tendency. These theorists hold that women become subordinate as a result of the interaction between the way work is organized and the way society is reproduced, a process that ceates social hierarchies of race, class, and gender. Forms of subordination differ from one economic organization to another; for example, women are restricted differently in agricultural, industrial, and pastoral societies. Feminist materialists influenced by Marx add a historical dimension to their analysis in order to understand the subordination of women at specific times in specific societies. Several first world feminists work cross culturally to obtain their insights or to explore the application of their ideas to third world societies. A number of third world feminists—for example, Nawal El Saadawi and Awa Thiam—adapt this set of lenses to examine women's condition in their society.

Women's health and health care can be analyzed in both of these theoretical frameworks but with different results. Although they take a social scientist's view, writers adopting the psychological approach to women's health emphasize biological aspects of women's experience such as pregnancy and childbirth. Those who take a materialist stance view women's health problems as socially constructed or economically determined. Social psychologists of gender say that women's poor health stems from the subordination of women in patriarchal/capitalist societies, and that poor health care is delivered by a medical corps dominated by men with sexist attitudes who apply medical theories developed by male thinkers in economies oriented to profit-making. Political economists of health say that social relations of production and forces of production determine general levels of health and health services for men and women, but women's health is additionally affected by gender relations within the social relations of production as well as by the conditions of reproduction, which include the availability of maternal health services (Turshen 1989).

The concept of women's subordination as used in this book differs from that of discrimination against women. Subordination refers to relations of gender and to male dominance of those relations, not to biologically determined roles or functions. Subordination also refers to the gender and class relations that derive from the economic organization of society. Subordination is a dynamic concept, and it is historically specific. In this framework, women's ill health reflects both men's continuing domination of women and changing economic relations such as new sexual divisions of labor, new forms of production, and changing conditions of reproduction.

In outline, the book opens with a description of the impact of war on women's health in Mozambique. The following four chapters deal with aspects of women's productive work on plantations, in nursing, in domestic work, and in trading and subsistence farming. A general theoretical chapter on gender and health effects a transition from the discussion of productive labor to a consideration of women's reproductive work. The concluding chapter sketches women's health care needs. Each chapter is described in detail below.

The War on Women

In Chapter Two, Julie Cliff describes the war on women in Mozambique and the impact of destabilization and structural adjustment on women's health. Cliff describes a nation under a double attack: on one side, an internationally financed army of bandits wreaks havoc on the country's economic and social infrastructure and destroys the psychological and physical security of a society; and on the other side, international organizations dictate fiscal policies which, instead of enabling the country to rebuild its damaged infrastructure, further undermine health and educational services. These policies are designed to turn the government away from socialist development. RENAMO, the antigovernment force, and the International Monetary Fund (IMF) are symbols of a deeper crisis engendered partly by South Africa's policies of economic, political, and military destabilization of the region and partly by the critical state of African economies.

Immediately after independence, Mozambicans saw advances in women's health care. The primary health care network expanded rapidly and trained many women health workers. The result was better access to basic health services for increasing numbers of women. Since 1982, women's health in Mozambique has suffered as South African destabilization forced the closure of peripheral maternity units and disrupted rural life. As part of a structural adjustment program, introduced in 1987, the government has withdrawn food subsidies and increased health service charges.

Mozambique is a worst case scenario but it is not unique in Africa. In the 1980s civil wars were fought in Angola, Chad, Ethiopia, Sudan, Uganda, and the Western Sahara with varying amounts of outside influence. And the IMF imposed its draconian solutions on a majority of sub-Saharan governments. UNICEF alone among the international organizations has traced the impact of war and "structural adjustment" (the IMF's euphemism for its fiscal imperatives) on children and their mothers.

As Cliff shows, the first condition for women's health is peace, for without personal security no one can preserve the material gains of their labor. The second condition is food security. Without it, the need to assure subsistence becomes a fulltime preoccupation, especially for women who supply most or all of the food eaten in the household. A third condition is gainful employment.

The Impact of Productive Labor on Women's Health

Because industrialization is so limited in sub-Saharan Africa and because women are so underrepresented in industrial employment, studies of African women in paid employment are rare. Yet African women increasingly find paid work, often in conditions that are less than ideal (OIT 1985). In the Joliba cigarette factory of Mali, women comprise more than one-third of the workforce; hours are strict and employers make no concessions for the difficulties of transport, child care, or family meal preparation (Condé 1983, 113). In Senegal, as in other sub-Saharan countries, women workers are concentrated in the food and textile industries. A fluctuating workforce of day and seasonal laborers, Senegalese women work under difficult conditions without social benefits such as a minimum wage (Savané 1983, 115).

Women's occupational health is even less studied than women's employment; René Loewenson's study of women at work on Zimbabwean plantations therefore fills an important gap. Industrial health is in general an understudied subject in Africa (Turshen 1986). Most research focuses on mining, in keeping with Amin's (1989) observation that Africa's interest for the West is its mineral wealth. Surveys of occupational health in the agricultural sector, including plantations, are almost non-existent. Yet most Africans, and especially most women, work on farms, and plantations are a feature of agricultural production in Côte d'Ivoire, Kenya, Malawi, Senegal, South Africa, Tanzania, and Zimbabwe, to name but a few sites.

Loewenson describes the socioeconomic status of labor in the private large-scale farm sector in Zimbabwe, drawing from both original field data and secondary sources. She highlights the specific nature and status of women's labor within the general context of production relations. She places particular emphasis on the past decade, when shifts toward increasing capital intensity of production (the use of machines and chemicals) resulted in declining plantation employment and greater recourse to casual seasonal labor, often female. She describes the impact on women's socioeconomic status of common employment practices such as the piece wage system.

Because she does not see women as passive, Loewenson explores the sociopolitical status of women's labor. She analyzes local government, trade union, party, and state structures to determine the extent to which they empower women to change the factors that condition their health. Loewenson examines the health impact of plantation employment and environmental and social conditions on women and children. She discusses the nature of health services on plantations, the role of women as health care providers, and workers' struggle for health in general.

Health and education are two major categories of women's work in Africa. Most positions in health and education are public sector jobs; between them, these ministries employ most women workers. In Senegal, 66 percent of female government employees work for these two ministries; in Madagascar the figure is 73 percent (OIT 1985, 82). Women account for 30 percent of health ministry employees in Madagascar and 40 percent of workers in the ministry of education. In Senegal, women workers account for 33 percent of government employees in health and 23 percent of employees in education. In Togo the figure is 42 percent in health; in Benin it is 38 percent (ibid.).

In South Africa as elsewhere, nurses form the largest group of health care providers, and the nursing service is essential to the nation's health. Nonceba Lubanga traces the combative history of black nurses' organizations under apartheid. Transcriptions of interviews with eyewitnesses enliven her account of the strikes organized by black nurses to improve patient care and their own working conditions.

Lubanga believes that as health advocates for patients, nurses have a moral obligation to identify and challenge the basic causes of inequalities in South African health services. She criticizes the compliant attitude of the white-dominated South African Nursing Council (SANC) and the South African Nursing Association (SANA); their passive acceptance of the regime and the injustices perpetrated against hospitalized victims of police and army violence are matters of grave concern. Under the emergency laws, which were recently repealed in some provinces, nurses and hospital administrators were instructed to keep a list of patients with bullet and buckshot wounds for police records and to cooperate with the government. Lubanga maintains that nurses cannot provide adequate care to their patients in the presence of intimidating military and police forces, now a familiar sight in the corridors and wards of most black hospitals in South Africa.

A third area of women's paid employment in Africa is domestic work. In the colonial period, European civil servants and industrialists hired African men to do housework, childcare, cooking, and gardening. Most Europeans departed at independence, but in the past thirty years, there has been increasing class differentiation among Africans, especially in urban areas, and the growing African bourgeoisie has replaced Europeans as employers of domestics.

Domestic work is now a predominantly female activity in Africa, but firm statistics are lacking on the numbers engaged in this socially devalued and economically undervalued occupation. Part of the huge influx of famished rural families into cities that lack an industrial base capable of absorbing a growing workforce (Amin 1989), many women take menial jobs as domestics in the hope that they will later find work in a factory. For many, the temporary situation becomes permanent, a phenomenon that is very common in Senegal (OIT 1985, 67).

Conditions of domestic work are deplorable—an enormous quantity of daily work is compensated by a derisory sum of money, and the younger the women, the less they are paid, although the quantity of work is not reduced correspondingly. Illiterate women are preferred because they are more docile, obedient, and less demanding. There are so many women offering their services in African cities and towns, and their situation is so critical, that every salaried worker can employ a domestic and pay her less than the minimum wage. Most countries have legislation that regulates domestic work, but it is rarely applied (ibid.).

Quarraisha Khan describes the health conditions of domestic workers in South Africa. Domestic service accounts for the employment of 38 percent of black women in South Africa. Roughly 89 percent of domestic servants are black and of these about 88 percent are women. Their conditions of work are the least protected within one of the most regimented labor forces in the world. Black domestic workers who live in their employers' homes are not allowed to bring their children to live with them. They may be separated from their families for days or months at a time, which as Khan shows through the story of Nonkululeko, causes them great anxiety about their children's welfare and deprives them of a normal married life. Khan examines the effects of such stress on women's health in this often humiliating occupation. She discusses the new trend, which has emerged in the past ten years, to unionize. Domestic workers in South Africa, as in Senegal, are beginning to organize and join trade unions in order to improve their working conditions.

A fourth category of women's work in Africa is trading. Throughout West Africa, women are well known as marketers engaged in both short- and long-distance trading. Most are self-employed, and the majority rarely earn enough to hire labor. At best they can rely on family help. Market women do not necessarily produce the products that they sell. In the past, the sexual division of labor in Nigeria, Ghana, and other West African countries, gave men the work of farming and women that of trading, but the current economic crisis seems to be causing a shift in these patterns.

Saba Mebrahtu collected ethnographic data on the changing nature of women's work in Nigeria. She found that women traders are being forced into farming, which is affecting household diets and the nutritional welfare of women and children. Formerly, Yoruba-speaking women rarely participated in any phase of agriculture because, they say, farming demands too much energy from a woman and causes her to age faster. But recently, Mebrahtu found, economic pressures forced more men to migrate from their farms, obliging their wives to take up subsistence farming in order to supplement or supply the family food budget. Reluctant to go into farming full time, these women adopt a cropping pattern that requires less time and energy; they are planting cassava, which is less labor intensive than yam production. Unfortunately the shift from yams to cassava leads to poorer nutrition for women and children because cassava has a lower protein content than yams.

Agricultural production is by far the largest category of work in Africa, but few women, other than plantation workers such as those described by Loewenson, are paid for their labor. At best, some are self-employed in the sense that they trade their produce and retain the profits. Many observers assume that there is a natural division of labor in sub-Saharan Africa, that the work women do is related to or compatible with their childbearing and child rearing functions. Roberts (1988) questions the naturalist model in terms of the allocation of labor in West African households: women's work patterns are dictated by their inability to mobilize the labor of others rather than by their ability to combine productive and domestic work. Why should it be natural for a woman in the last trimester of pregnancy carrying an additional twenty or more pounds, or a mother with a baby weighing as much as twenty-six pounds strapped to her back, to labor in the fields for up to ten hours a day? Is the implication that it is unnatural for men who are unencumbered by similar burdens to undertake this backbreaking work?

The chapter on gender and health bridges the two sections of the book with a discussion of the sexual politics of women's productive and reproductive labor. The key references to this theoretical discussion are Stichter and Parpart's introduction to *Patriarchy and Class: African Women in the Home and the Workforce* and a 1989 paper by Caldwell, Caldwell, and Quiggin entitled, "Disaster in an Alternative Civilization: The Social Dimensions of Aids in Sub-Saharan Africa." In the chapter, three questions are raised: who controls women's productive and reproductive labor, how is that control maintained, and how do women accept or evade control?

Reproductive Labor and Women's Health

Malika Ladjali created and directed for fifteen years the first family planning program in Algeria. She describes the opposition she encountered—from medical colleagues, who resisted the new powers given to midwives who were to deliver the services; from midwives, who were trained in clinical practice and resisted the public health orientation of the program; and from women, who rejected the idea of contraception or were afraid to come forward for the service. With training, health personnel changed their perspective. The more difficult obstacle proved to be the attitude of couples themselves. Ladjali recounts the study she undertook with Claudine Chaulet of the demand for contraception and the conclusions they reached on who controls women's fertility, how that control is maintained, and in which circumstances it can be renegotiated. Ladjali also describes the evaluation she undertook of the Algerian family planning program and the changes made as a result.

In 1986, the objectives of the Algerian program changed when the government decided that the birth rate, which was thirty-nine live births per thousand population, was higher than what the economy could support. As Jenny Lindsay shows in the chapter on

Namibia, the impact of population control on women's health is very different from that of family planning.

Population control in Namibia has always been central to South African strategies of administration in this former colonial territory. The colonial government maintained control of the population by means of contracts under the migrant labor system, by the confinement of black Namibians to reserves and separate residential areas in towns, and by the requirement of passes. Today, however, contraceptive technology facilitates yet another method of control, the direct regulation of black women's fertility. The government instituted a family planning program in hospitals and clinics throughout Namibia. This program, which uses Depo-Provera (an injectable hormonal contraceptive) and forced sterilizations to bring down birth rates, manifests the violent nature of the South African state. Lindsay documents the implementation of this family planning program by the state and by the white ruling classes, and also the resistance to it. She analyzes population control in terms of class, race, and gender relations in Namibia, rather than as simply yet another example of oppression (though it is that too). She sees control over reproduction as a question of struggle, and the resistance of black Namibians to state policies as part of the ongoing struggle for independence.

Lindsay bases her findings on research that she carried out between 1983 and 1986. She used anthroplogical methods and gathered oral evidence in interviews with Namibian women and Namibian physicians. The political situation dictated the choice of these methods. Lack of significant documentary evidence and meaningful statistical data has handicapped all research projects in Namibia. The rapid approach of independence, which was finally celebrated March 21, 1990, gave an importance to even tentative and exploratory findings. Lindsay hopes that her work will be of some use in suggesting avenues for more rigorous investigation in independent Namibia, because birth control policies are of vital importance for Namibian women.

Crude birth rates of 39 per 1,000 population (Algeria), 45 per 1,000 population (Namibia) and 51 per 1,000 population (Côte d'Ivoire) are typical of Africa. Total fertility [1] tops off at six, seven, or eight children per woman. How do African women cope?

Agnès Guillaume gives one answer in a discussion of the West African practice of fostering children. In Côte d'Ivoire, total fertility was 7.4 children in 1987. If a woman were to raise all of her children in the fifteen to twenty year period in which they are born, her time would be almost completely occupied by childcare. To free themselves for other work, which Guillaume shows is very varied with each woman undertaking multiple tasks, Ivorian women arrange for a family member such as a grandmother who may have no access to labor, to foster one or more of their children. Fostering lightens the burden of child rearing and reduces household expenses at a critical time in the family's growth. These same women, at a later stage of their lives when their children are grown, may in turn foster one or more children. Guillaume asks what effect this practice has on the health of mothers and children and what arrangements women can make for their own and their children's health care.

The final country case study examines the impact of a new disease, AIDS, on women in Zaire. The epidemic, which in Africa is killing equal numbers of women and men, offers a peculiar—macabre—opportunity to study the effects of patriarchy on disease control.

There has been no dearth of pronouncements on the liberation of women in Zaire, but the reality remains patriarchal. By law everyone has the right to work and sexual discrimination is forbidden, but no woman can obtain a commercial license or open a bank account without her husband's authorization (MacGaffey 1988, 163). Women are generally relegated to underpaid work and jobs can be obtained only through social connections or by accepting the boss' sexual advances. If a woman becomes pregnant, she loses one-third of her salary (Lanza 1983, 132).

Faced with these difficulties, many women are forced to depend on husbands or lovers. Monogamy is the rule in Zaire, but irregular forms of polygamy are common and tolerated. Unmarried women attached to married men are referred to as "*deuxième bureaux*"—as in, "Don't expect me for dinner, honey, I'm working late at the office." Even high school girls are caught up in these arrangements, which enable them to finish their studies or help support their families.

It is easy to confuse this situation with prostitution and to imagine, in the generalized corruption of Mobutu's Zaire where "everything is for sale" (ibid.), that women have no protection against rape or abandonment. Girls receive no sexual education in school. Although the Pill is freely sold, supplies are difficult to obtain. Abortion is illegal, and illegal abortion is common.

The outbreak of the AIDS epidemic gives a new and sinister meaning to this behavior. Brooke Grundfest Schoepf, Walu Engundu, Rukarangira wa Nkera, Payanzo ntsomo, and Claude Schoepf worked with Zairian women in a project called CONNAISSIDA teaching them ways to protect themselves against AIDS. They found an understanding of culturally constructed gender roles and sexual meanings to be crucial to the development of disease control measures. AIDS assumed epidemic proportions in Central Africa during a period of prolonged economic crisis. Policies promulgated to promote economic stabilization have exacerbated poverty, particularly among women. Women and children together constitute the greatest number of persons affected by AIDS. By linking macrolevel political economy to microlevel sociocultural analysis, Schoepf and her coauthors show how the strategies that women adopted for survival have turned into death strategies.

Virtually the entire adult population of Kinshasa is aware that AIDS is incurable, lethal, and transmitted by sexual relations. As in many other parts of the world, however, few of those at risk have actually changed their behavior; the psychological mechanisms of denial and avoidance keep them from recognizing their vulnerability. Gendered and class structured social relations impede the adoption of protective behavior. The authors used medical anthropology and experiential training to develop culturally appropriate, community-based, risk reduction workshops, which employ cognitive, emotional, and social stimulants.

The AIDS epidemic raises fundamental questions about the health care strategies of African governments and the bilateral and multilateral aid agencies on which they are dependent. Instead of developing basic health services, donors are distributing condoms to prevent the spread of the AIDS virus. The consequences for African women are devastating.

The concluding chapter explores the relation of gender to health by focusing on the social production of women's health care. Like women's health status, women's health services develop within specific political economies. In Africa, two forces conditioned the post-independence political economies: colonialism, which differed from one country to another even within the same empire, and indigenous political structures, which had been transformed by the colonial experience. Colonial health services were especially marked by metropolitan models. After independence governments followed varied development paths, and plans for the expansion of health services were correspondingly diverse. The one constant appears to be inadequate health care for women.

Feminist work within the theoretical framework of the subordination of women shows that the level and type of service offered to women are tied to women's economic and political power. Because women command less power than men, women's health care is rarely of the same quality or of equal technical sophistication as the care offered to men. Although the care available to the population is generally conditioned by the economic limits and political possibilities of governments, women's health services vary significantly according to the control women have of their productive and reproductive labor; and that control is a function of women's economic, social, and political participation in society. Women's ability to express their interests politically is predictive of whether women control definitions of health and illness, whether health care is adapted to their needs, and whether they have access to health services. These points are illustrated with the example of women's reproductive health care.

· 2 ·

The War on Women in Mozambique

Health Consequences of South African Destabilization, Economic Crisis, and Structural Adjustment

JULIE CLIFF

JOANA C. lay, weighing just 99 pounds, in the respiratory diseases ward of Maputo Central Hospital. She was seriously ill, her body weakened by nine months of insufficient food, and her lungs damaged by tuberculosis. Although she was recovering, she still did not see how she could manage when she went home. Since basic food prices rose sharply nine months before, she had been barely able to feed her children adequately, let alone herself.

Although her salary as a domestic employee had risen, the increase was less than the price rises. She now had to put extra time and energy into her other source of income, selling chewing gum, and she was still too weak. Fortunately, she had her eleven-year-old niece who had come to the city to help with the children. A pity they had not been able to afford schooling for the niece, as they had originally intended. She was afraid her husband would leave her. After all, who wanted a sick wife; her first husband had abandoned her after their two children died. At least she now had healthy children by this husband.

It seemed as if things could not get worse. But they did; two weeks after her discharge from hospital Joana C. was back again, this time with her six-year-old daughter, Maria, who lay in a coma induced by cerebral malaria. After discharge from hospital, Maria was blind, deaf, and needed fulltime care, so Joana C. was forced to stop work to care for her. Only time would tell if the brain damage was permanent.

Joana C. is one of the women who benefited from Mozambique's new health services, introduced after independence in 1975. Before independence, she had lost her two children, one to measles, the other to neonatal tetanus. Her own tuberculosis had been only partly treated; she stopped treatment after only two months because she felt better. The tuberculosis recurred in 1983; this time she completed the treatment course. After independence, she raised four healthy children, taking them regularly for weighing and immunizations. She began to use contraceptives, first an intrauterine device to space her third and fourth children, and then Depo-Provera. She also attended literacy classes, although she dropped out when the classes became too difficult and she was pregnant with her fifth child.

Joana C.'s family suffered directly because of the war that grinds on in the country's rural areas. Bandits of the South African-backed RENAMO (Mozambique National Resistance) sabotage economic targets and terrorize civilians in their campaign to topple the Mozambican government. They wounded or kidnapped many of Joana C.'s close relatives and had burnt all the family homes to the ground, forcing them all to flee to the safety of the city, often expecting to share her meager resources. Two of her children had been in the care of her mother in her home area; after their school was destroyed, depriving them of schooling, and all their clothes were burnt, they too had fled to the city.

The impact of the government's economic reform program had been sharp. With the price rises, the family was unable to live on their joint salaries; her husband earned less than the minimum wage as a guard. They could survive only by borrowing money.

They had to move from their small cement dwelling near the city center to a hastily constructed reed hut on the outskirts. She felt too weak to walk the four miles to and from work. The suburb was served only by expensive private transport and the journey lasted one hour each way, leaving her less time for other work. Her children suffered frequent illnesses after the move. She often could not afford the increased cost of the prescribed drugs at the local health center, so she had to borrow more money to buy them. Both she and her daughter, however, received free hospital treatment for their latest illnesses; without this treatment their chances of survival would have been small.

Helena M. is the chief nurse in the surgical unit of Houlene Hospital in Maputo. A strong, competent woman, she talks to me about how she came to her present job and the impact of the war on her family. She has just four years of schooling. Even this was remarkable for the colonial period (in 1970 only 2 percent of Africans over six years old had completed four years of primary education, most of them men). She was one of five children in a rural peasant family. At age six, her older brother, a school teacher in the local Catholic mission, gave her over to the care of the nuns. At age twelve, she went to the capital for schooling; after four years she had to stop, as there was no money to continue. So she trained as an auxiliary midwife, the only category open to blacks. Whites received a higher status and salary as nurse midwives. After independence, nurses were in short supply, as Portuguese nurses left and the health services expanded. Her obvious competence led to rapid promotion; in 1983, she studied for a full year to be a chief nurse.

As we talk, her elderly father comes into the room. I am shocked to see him; formerly a spry man, he is now visibly dejected and emaciated. I assume he is sick, but he is recovering after the bandits displaced him from his home for a second time. His wife is still in their place of refuge; he is anxious to get back, although his daughter wants them to come to Maputo. Their place of refuge is not fertile; the soil is not good enough to grow peanuts, their main protein source. Also, many people are crowded together. The nearest water source is 1.5 miles away; the nearest health post is at their first place of refuge, 1.8 miles distant. The bandits have attacked the post many times, the last time the previous month.

Access to the post for women in labor is now severely limited; travel at night is too dangerous, and the midwife is too frightened to sleep close to the maternity unit, a target for the bandits. Helena M. thinks that women are more vulnerable than men in this war; the bandits are more likely to kidnap them, as women's daily tasks of cultivation and water collection oblige them to travel in the bush. Once kidnapped, women are more likely to be killed unless they are young and not pregnant.

Serena T. sits lifelessly. She does not want to eat, she cannot sleep, and she cannot see what she is going to do with her life. Nothing is worth doing. Two months earlier she was a heroine, having made a courageous escape after capture by RENAMO. She was director of health services in a remote border district and was captured in the hospital trenches with her patients during a RENAMO attack. Knowing the fate that awaited her if she were recognized, she had pretended to be a patient; the women patients had willingly helped her assume this disguise. She had escaped during the long march to the bandits' base, and ran all the way back to the town, now retaken by Government troops. She found the hospital and her house destroyed; all her belongings were gone.

She was among the first groups trained as medical assistants in the capital; her course gave her competence in a wide range of preventive and curative skills. The last part of the practical training was in the remote northern province of Niassa; afterwards, a group volunteered to stay on. She is now too frightened to return, and wants to go to the capital in her home province of Zambezia.

These three stories illustrate some post-independence successes in women's health in Mozambique: a woman with tuberculosis and her children receiving improved health care, and the opening up of educational opportunities for women health workers. In recent years, South African destabilization has eroded the gains. All three women have suffered; Serena T. most dramatically by kidnapping, Helena M. and Joana C. by separation from their families in the rural areas. Joana C., the domestic employee without a profession, suffered most from the economic reforms imposed by structural adjustment policies; she could no longer feed her family adequately. Desperate as the current situation is, it still is an improvement over the colonial years.

Mozambican women's lives under Portuguese colonialism were characterized by exploitation. With the emigration of male laborers, particularly to the South African mines, men's work burdens were taken over by the women who stayed behind; the forced cultivation of cash crops was added to the normal burden of producing the family food supply. The Portuguese also forced women to labor for them; women built most of Mozambique's roads. Diet and fertility were depressed; vulnerability to epidemic diseases increased (Kruks and Wisner 1984, 113). In the capital city, Maputo, a huge prostitution industry thrived, based on South African tourists and visiting seamen.

Women had few opportunities for education, and colonial health services for them were rudimentary. For example, at independence in 1975, the overall illiteracy rate was 90 percent; for women, it was even higher. There were only seven antenatal clinics, all in urban areas, for a population of ten million.

Changes Since Independence

Stephanie Urdang (1989) has vividly documented the changes brought to women's lives by independence. The new government abolished forced labor, forced cultivation, and the tourist trade in prostitutes. Education and literacy expanded; primary enrollment went from 600,000 to 1,600,000 in five years and the illiteracy rate fell from 90 percent to 72 percent (Marshall 1988). A sexual differential persisted; the rate for women was 85 percent, compared to 59 percent for men. Also, the sexual division of labor within the household remained unchanged, limiting women's possibilities for increased leisure, education, and work outside the home.

Women gained many new rights. For example, the government granted two months' maternity leave at full pay, facilitating women's entry into the workforce, and passed new legislation to encourage women to breastfeed their infants.

In 1977, the government created a national health service; health care was provided for a token charge. Women gained increased access to health services as the primary health care network expanded rapidly, from 426 units in 1975 to 1,171 in 1982. The platform of the ruling party, FRELIMO, at the third party congress in 1977 gave priority to maternal and child health services. A commitment of resources accompanied the rhetoric; maternity beds increased by 30 percent (2,680 to 3,610) between 1975 and 1986, compared with an overall expansion of hospital beds of 20 percent. The number of midwives increased from 457 in 1980 to 971 in 1986. Between 1979 and 1981, routine data showed that, nationally, the percentage of women attending antenatal clinics had increased from 40 percent to 49 percent. The percentage delivering in maternity units rose from 27 to 29 percent.

The government introduced family planning services. Recognizing the need to avoid a vertical program, the health ministry integrated family planning within the maternal and child health services. The ministry also integrated clinics for mothers with those for children, enabling mothers to take care of theirs and their children's health needs in a single visit.

Health workers' treatment of women improved, as democratization of the health services after independence gave patients more rights (Walt and Melamed 1984). Midwives had often treated women in labor harshly; in 1976, wide publicity was given to the sacking of Katija, a cleaner in Maputo Central Hospital's maternity unit, notorious for her sadistic abuse of women in labor.

Training of women health workers increased. Many women chose to train as doctors; 52 percent of the students in the University Medical Faculty are women. Only two women, however, have risen to the level of National Director in the Ministry of Health hierarchy, both in the traditional women's field of social action.

Most village health workers have been men, as the selection process demanded four years of primary education, rare in women at village level. Women, however, did not accept male village health workers as attendants during delivery; therefore, in 1984, training courses for female traditional birth attendants began.

South African Destabilization

Destabilization of Mozambique began soon after independence, as the security services of Ian Smith's Rhodesia (now Zimbabwe) threw resources into a Mozambican rebel movement they had created, the Mozambique National Resistance (RENAMO). Mozambique was then providing a rear base for ZANU, the movement fighting for Zimbabwe's independence. When ZANU gained power in 1980 the South Africans took over RENAMO, relocating the rebels in South Africa. In 1982, RENAMO attacks within Mozambique began again; they have continued ever since. The targets are the economic infrastructure, the civilian population, and the visible government successes of health and education facilities.

Women have been direct victims of RENAMO. Attention has focused on child abuse by RENAMO (Summerfield 1988:8590); less attention has been paid to the abuse of women. While RENAMO has brutalized their children, training them as killers, mothers have endured rape and life as chattels of RENAMO. Gersony (1988) has described life under RENAMO from refugee accounts. Over 15 percent of those interviewed "reported patterns of systematic rape of civilian women by RENAMO combatants." In areas controlled by RENAMO, a

> function of the young girls and women is to provide sex for the combatants ... these women are required to submit to sexual demands, in effect to be raped, on a frequent, sustained basis.... One of the frequent refugee complaints (verified by medical workers in some of the refugee camps) is the level of infection with venereal diseases which this practice proliferates. Severe beating is

inflicted on young girls and women who resist sexual demands. Such punishment may also be inflicted on the husband or father of the female who resists. Such punishment reportedly can include execution in some circumstances.

With RENAMO attacks, rural women's lives have become increasingly insecure. The migrant labor system left women as the tenders of family farms in the rural areas. In addition to the long hours spent producing the family food supply, they now have to spend time in a search for safety, often sleeping the night in the bush with their children, as RENAMO attacks usually occur after dark. A trip to collect water becomes a perilous journey, as bandits may be lying in wait. Many women have fled their homes and fields, some to towns and cities, others to safer rural areas. By April 1989, an estimated 1,600,000 people had been displaced within Mozambique.

In the cities, life for women became increasingly difficult, as the war induced an economic crisis. Widespread shortages of goods resulted; a parallel market with exorbitant prices thrived. For example, wood and charcoal prices soared because, as the population increased, the forest margins retreated, and transport networks broke down. In 1986, the real salary in Maputo was estimated to be only 16.5 percent of its value in 1981, while for the country as a whole it was 31 percent (Francisco et al. 1987, 17). Urban women have always moved back and forth to the rural areas. As wages were never sufficient to support a family, sale of produce from the family farm provided a necessary supplement. War disrupted this pattern, forcing women to abandon their farms and to seek other sources of income in the city.

Direct information on the impact of the war on women's health is scarce. Reduced access to maternity units for delivery has undoubtedly increased maternal deaths from hemorrhages, infections, eclampsia, and anemia. Information is available on childhood malnutrition and, generally, when children are malnourished, women (who provide their food) also suffer nutritional deficiencies.

Childhood nutrition surveys in 1988 showed wide variations in malnutrition rates. For example, in Cabo Delgado province, less affected by war, the mean acute malnutrition rate in children under five years old was 4.9 percent. However, in one group of children displaced by war the rate was 20 percent. In a severely affected part of Zambezia province, the rate reached 48 percent. Where food supplies were adequate, lower rates were recorded (Secçao de Nutriçao 1989). Mothers have seen their children's health worsen with the war, as they fell victim to malnutrition and infectious diseases. A report for the United Nations Children's Fund (UNICEF 1989, 25) estimates that, between 1980 and 1988, the war caused 494,000 excess deaths in children.

In the only study of adult malnutrition, Ramji (1987) showed that the proportion of severe malnutrition among elderly Mozambican women (women over forty-five years of age) in centers for the displaced was 21 percent, using a weight of under 40 kilograms as a cutoff point; it was 9 percent, using a body mass index (weight over height squared) of under 15. The corresponding percentages for men were 5 percent and 2 percent.

The war has destroyed much of the fabric of Mozambican society. Women have lost their husbands and been separated from their children. No comprehensive figures are available on the number of women widowed by the war. In July 1987, in one center for displaced persons in Tete province, sixty-one war widows were registered out of a total population of 1,141. In Ramji's survey of elderly displaced women in centers, 64 percent in Mozambique and 74 percent in Zimbabwe were widows (1987, 13).

RENAMO has targeted the health and education services (Cliff and Noormahomed 1988; Marshall 1988). In the education sector, the war caused the closure of 2,269 primary schools, depriving more than 500,000 children of classes. In the health sector between 1982 and 1987, 822 health units were destroyed or forced to close. Maternity units have come under direct attack: for example, in Inhambane province, attendance at maternity units for delivery dropped after a massacre in the town of Homoine, when RENAMO bandits murdered pregnant women who were waiting to deliver in the hospital. In Maputo, peripheral maternity units now close at night following a series of bandit attacks and kidnappings. The previous increase in attendance has been halted; nationally, routine data show that the percentage of women attending antenatal clinics fell from 49 percent in 1981 to 45 percent in 1986. The percentage attending maternity units for delivery fell from 29 percent to 27 percent over the same period.

Women health workers have also been direct victims. Bandits have kidnapped many from their workplaces, making them frightened to work in isolated war-affected districts. A new program to train large numbers of young women as maternal and child health workers was planned to improve the quality of maternal and child health care in the rural areas. But the program ran into difficulties, as newly trained workers are reluctant to move away from provincial capitals.

Economic Crisis and Structural Adjustment

In 1987, Mozambique began a series of structural adjustments to its economic policy, announcing an economic reform program. By then, the country was in the midst of perhaps the worst economic crisis in Africa (Loxley 1988, 3). The estimated losses from war totalled over U.S.$5.5 billion, more than the country's external debt, and sixty times the value of 1987 exports (Gabriel 1988). Although the war was the overwhelming cause, other factors contributed: a dependence on primary product exports in an inequitable world trading system, an extreme shortage of managerial personnel, and early policy errors that gave priority to state farms in agriculture (Munslow 1988). South Africa had also squeezed the Mozambican economy by cutting the numbers of mine workers and by diverting traffic from Mozambican to South African ports and railways.

The economic crisis took the form of a collapse of production and trade, resulting in shortages of essential goods, inflation, parallel markets, a foreign exchange shortage, and an inability to balance the government budget. By 1986, export earnings from merchandise were only U.S.$34 million, 28 percent of their 1980 level. Mozambique serviced its debt only up to 1982; by 1986, the outstanding external debt had risen to U.S.$3.4 billion, completely beyond servicing (Hermele 1988, 11).

Economic reform was necessary. A massive inflow of foreign exchange and a rescheduling of debt commitments needed to restore production were dependent on agreements with the International Monetary Fund and the World Bank (Loxley 1988, 5). The reforms include massive devaluation of the Mozambican currency, the meticai, and an opening to market forces. The currency has been progressively devalued, falling from a value of forty-two meticais to one U.S. dollar in early 1987 to a ratio of 620:1 in October 1988. The government cut public expenditure, most severely in health and education, and introduced or increased fees in these sectors. Subsidies were reduced or removed, leading to price increases in staple food, rents, and utilities. Although salaries were also raised, increases repeatedly lagged behind price rises.

In April 1988, most staple food prices suddenly rose by 400 to 600 percent, as the government removed food subsidies. Previously, food for urban consumers had been heavily subsidized. Donors provide most food in Mozambique because internal production is so low; for example, 90 percent of cereals were donated in 1989. The United States and other large donors require Mozambique to pay the local currency value of sold food into an account that can be drawn upon only with donor consent. With the removal of subsidies, costs were passed on to urban consumers, who now have to pay the high U.S. grain prices in a country where the minimum wage is less than U.S.$30 per month (Hanlon 1988).

The economic reform program was initially successful in restoring economic growth. In 1987, the overall growth rate was 3.7 percent, the first increase since 1981. An abundance of goods appeared in previously empty shops, transforming the appearance of the urban centers. The volume of goods marketed by peasants increased by 27 percent and industrial output by 18 percent. The International Monetary Fund has cautioned, however, that growth will probably not be sustainable in the short run, although it maintains that conditions for medium and long-term growth are improved (Hermele 1988, 18).

Some economists question the sustainability of growth in a war situation, when there is no efficient market solution to reestablishing the economy (Hermele 1988, 19; Loxley 1988, 5; Mackintosh 1986, 575; Wuyts 1989, 22). Also, in a country at war, economic activity needs to be organized to support the war effort. No country has prosecuted a war on its own territory, with mobilization of the whole population, without establishing considerable state economic planning (Mackintosh 1986, 575).

No direct information is available on the impact of adjustment on women in Mozambique. It is therefore necessary to forward the theoretical case for a negative impact of adjustment on women, and then present the data showing the negative impact of adjustment on the urban poor in Mozambique.

Structural adjustment has an in-built gender bias against women. As Elson (1987, 3) shows,

> When macro-economic policies are formulated to reallocate resources, the lack of explicit consideration of the process of reproduction and human resources tells against women. For the implicit assumption of macro-economic policy is that the process of reproduction and maintenance of human resources which is carried out unpaid by women will continue regardless of the way in which resources are reallocated ... the success of the macro-economic policy in reaching its goals may be won at the cost of a longer and harder working day for women. This cost will be invisible to the macro-economic policy makers because it is unpaid time. But the cost will be revealed in statistics on the health and nutritional status of such women.

Among the urban poor, women are a particularly vulnerable group during adjustment, as they tend to be in low-wage, low-status jobs and have few skills for wage employment. Particularly vulnerable are female heads of households.

Women's ability to promote health and nutrition for themselves and their families is conditioned by income, time, and education (Leslie, Lycette, and Buvinic 1986, 30). Adjustment usually reduces women's incomes. As formal sector employment opportunities for women are limited, adjustment forces them into lower-paying and less productive informal sector work (op. cit., 16). With reduced income, women have to spend more time earning extra income for the family, hunting for bargains, making and mending at home rather than buying (Elson 1987, 24). The increased demands on time potentially limit that available for health and nutrition-related activities. Girls and women are the first to drop out of school, as pressures increase for them to earn money and contribute their labor around the house. Female relatives have to substitute for mothers in child care.

The introduction of the economic reform program had a predictable negative social impact in urban areas of Mozambique. The currency devaluation and removal of subsidies caused sharp price rises that were not compensated for by wage increases. Urban poverty, therefore, increased and living standards declined, resulting in increased malnutrition.

Table 1 shows a comparison of wage and food price increases over 1987-89, using as an example the industrial minimum wage. The index of price increases substantially exceeded the index of wage increases. In Maputo and Beira, some basic foods, supplying approximately half of a person's caloric needs, are distributed through a rationing system. After most food subsidies were removed in April 1988, the cost of rationed food for a family of five was more than the minimum wage. To meet the costs of food, cooking fuel, transport, housing, health and education, a family would need at least two formal wage earners. Among female-headed households in Maputo city (21.7 percent of the total), 51.2 percent have no regularly employed member. Informal sector incomes probably also rose less rapidly than prices.

A survey in Maputo in August 1988 provided details of the impact of the economic reform program on individual families. Almost 82 percent of family expenses were on food and on energy to prepare food. Only 41.5 percent of the families took home all their food entitlement from the rationing system. The chronic malnutrition rate (low height for age) in children under five years old was 32.9 percent and the insufficient growth rate (no weight gain in two consecutive routine weighings) was 13.9 percent (Secçao de Nutriçao 1989). In June 1988, a similar survey in the provincial city of Tete showed a chronic malnutrition rate of 47.2 percent and an insufficient growth rate of 27 percent. Almost two-

TABLE 1
Wage and Price Increases in Mozambique,
1987-1989

	Jan. 1987	Jan. 1988	Jan. 1989
Minimum Wage (meticais/month)	2704	7500 (2.7)	17,000 (6.3)
Maize (meticais/kg)	9.0	27 (3.0)	112.5 (12.5)
Rice (meticais/kg)	13.5	40 (3.0)	271 (20.1)
Oil (meticais/ℓ)	58.5	630 (10.7)	630 (10.7)
Beans (meticais/kg)	27.0	195 (7.2)	260 (9.6)

Figures in brackets show the index compared to January 1987

thirds of the families had a per person income below 4,000 meticais, which is considered the minimum necessary for food security. In this group, 90 percent of families had children with insufficient growth (ibid.).

As studies on the impact of the economic reform program are urban-based, no information is available on rural areas. Rural households may be better off, as the economic reform program aims to benefit the rural areas at the expense of the urban. The impact of the war in rural areas, however, far outweighs the impact of the economic crisis, so any improvements in economic status will probably be marginal while the war continues.

In the health sector, expenditure was drastically cut, continuing a trend that began with the economic crisis. The percentage of the budget spent on health fell from 10.7 percent in 1981 to 4.4 percent in 1988. Inflation and devaluation have decreased the real value of expenditure on health from U.S.$4 per person in 1981 to less than five cents per person in 1988 (in constant 1980 meticais converted at prevailing exchange rates).

The economic crisis has led to an increased dependence on foreign aid to finance the health services. In 1987, the Mozambican government financed 47.3 percent, external aid financed 46.3 percent, and users financed 6.4 percent of recurrent health expenditure. External financing of drug imports was particularly high; in 1987 foreign sources financed almost 75 percent of total imports (Lopes-Valcarcel, Padron, Woodall, and Mello 1988, 13).

Donors and loan agencies, especially the large multilateral organizations such as the World Bank and UNICEF, now have increasing influence in health policymaking. A multiplicity of small organizations help in implementation. Funds tend to be allocated to projects, leading to a fragmentation of the primary health care approach. As the health minister cautioned: "We lose the sense of unity in our institutions when we replace programs with projects" (AIM 1989a).

The economic reform program included a rise in outpatient fees from 7.5 meticais to 100 meticais, and the introduction of an inpatient fee of 500 meticais in some hospitals. Employers must pay for employees' inpatient care; maternity patients and children are among a long list of groups exempted from charges. The aim of the increase was to improve the quality of care by allocating the fees collected to the health sector, and thus compensate for the drastic reductions in recurrent health expenditure in the government budget. Unfortunately, the higher charges created access barriers for the poorest. In Maputo's Cement City (the old settler area in the center of the city), outpatient visits fell by 23.5 percent from 1986 to 1987 and by 8.6 percent, from 1987 to 1988. In the poorer shanty towns outside the Cement City, the fall was 32.7 percent from 1986 to 1987, with a small improvement of 1.3 percent from 1987 to 1988. In one detailed study at a rural hospital, outpatient consultations dropped with the increase in fees; hospital deliveries, which remained free, showed only a slight drop (Krug 1988). Some health units registered increased attendance; others recovered after an initial fall.

Drug prices also rose, initially to cover the full cost of procurement and distribution. With further currency devaluations, the charges no longer covered costs. The price of many basic drugs to the consumer remained low; the estimated cost of a primary health care prescription in 1988 was 100-150 meticais. The cost of antibiotics, and drugs for some chronic illnesses, was prohibitively high, however. For example, for a family on the minimum wage, treatment of an episode of pneumonia would cost more than 11 percent of monthly income (Kanji 1989, 115). Some partial information is available on the impact of price rises on patient drug use. A study at Infulene Health Center in Maputo showed that 17 percent of outpatients were unable to afford the drug bill (average amount 635 meticais). In other provinces, 4 to 18 percent of outpatients did not buy prescribed drugs (Lopes-Valcarcel, Padron, Woodall, and Mello 1988).

In the first two years of operation, cost-recovery from the new drug charges was negligible. In 1987, actual collections for drugs were 4.6 percent of the value of allocations. On balance, the new charges contributed only marginally to revenue gains; any gains were offset by the increased amount of professional time involved in administration.

In the education sector, the economic reform program package included privatization of school materials and books; costs for each child are from 3,000 to 5,000 meticais per year, a sum beyond the means of poor families (Marshall 1989, 15). In 1988, an urban minimum wage earner spent 21 percent of his/her salary, and an agricultural minimum wage earner 35 percent, to maintain three children in school.

The economic reform program had a negative impact, therefore, on both the education and health services, leading one observer to caution that the shortterm financial gains of the economic reform program may well be offset by longterm reduced productivity owing to a deterioration of these services (Hermele 1988, 27).

Women health workers have been hit by the relative rise in prices compared with wages. Female heads of household are a particularly disadvantaged group during economic crisis and adjustment; many single women work in the health services as nurses and cleaners. Many health workers, both men and women, have had to seek other sources of income, spending less time in their health service jobs, with a resulting drop in the quality of care. Corruption tempts more workers, and pressures for privatization have increased.

In Mozambique, the social impact of adjustment has been monitored through the studies cited above, and with the assistance of WHO and UNICEF. UNICEF has been active internationally in pressing for monitoring of the social impact of structural adjustment on the vulnerable. More recently, the World Bank has begun a project on the social dimensions of adjustment, which aims to improve the capacity of member states in sub-Saharan Africa, including Mozambique, to monitor the impact of adjustment on the welfare of the poor. Clearly, independent monitoring is also necessary.

Most monitoring of the impact of adjustment has focused on families as a whole. In the future, women's health and economic status should also be monitored. The key issue is whether adjustment in fact works by increasing the amount of unpaid labor women have to do (Elson 1987, 5). To show the true cost to women of adjustment, studies must provide time budget data and nutrition and health status indicators. For women, monitoring of intrahousehold resource allocation is also crucial.

UNICEF recognizes the need to cushion the social impact of adjustment and is promoting the concept of "adjustment with a human face." In the early 1980s, international agencies considered the fate of vulnerable groups to be a matter for national governments to deal with, rather than an issue of adjustment policy. UNICEF now considers a broader approach necessary (Cornia, Jolly, and Stewart 1987).

The World Bank accepts the need for compensatory programs and is now assisting countries, including Mozambique, to implement them. In 1989, the Mozambican government introduced various compensatory measures, including a social fund for medicines and supplementary food for children. Medicines are now free for disadvantaged groups, and the chronically ill receive an 80 percent reduction in cost (AIM 1989a). The government also decided to reintroduce subsidies on certain foods, notably maize and rice, to cushion the impact of price rises on the urban poor (AIM 1989b).

Laudable though these attempts are, they entail a radical change in philosophy for Mozambique. Previously, the underlying social philosophy was a generalized system of meeting basic needs on the basis of need rather than ability to pay. Underlying the economic reform program is the acceptance of a two-tier economy. In the upper tier, effective demand (which is demand backed by income) determines access to consumer goods and services. In the lower tier, safety nets aim to protect vulnerable groups in the process of adjustment, and special programs provide for the targeted needs of the destitute (Wuyts 1989, 21).

Although some compensatory programs will cushion the impact on poor women, they are not specifically designed to benefit women. The concept of adjustment with a human face focuses on women as victims rather than on their potential contribution to effective adjustment (Elson 1987, 27). Strategies to ameliorate the impact of adjustment on women must aim to reduce time conflicts, increase women's incomes, and improve their education (Leslie, Lycette, and Buvinic 1986, 30). To lighten the burden of their unpaid work, women need the support of the public sector to provide water supplies, public transport, health care, and education. Women's interests lie, not in reducing the role of the state and increasing the role of the market, but in restructuring both the private and public sectors to make them more responsive to women's needs (Elson 1987, 14).

Elson (ibid., 28) suggests adjustment with gender equity, a policy requiring greater selectivity in public expenditure cuts, a restructuring of public sector activities, and a greater emphasis on self-reliant food production. It also requires more finance from donors to permit a slower pace of adjustment and provision of appropriate technical assistance and training.

External Changes

Adjustment focuses on internal policies. In Mozambique, however, the main cause of the economic crisis is external—South African destabilization. Removal of financial support from South Africa, the adoption of more economic sanctions against South Africa, and increased support for the frontline states are effective ways to hasten the end of the apartheid regime and to improve women's health in Mozambique.

The burden of adjustment is falling disproportionately on the poorest developing countries such as Mozambique; the rules of the game of the international economy are not being adjusted (ibid., 8).

Other economic changes, such as writing off debts and fairer prices for primary products on the world market, will also improve Mozambique's economy and women's health.

In conclusion, women's health in Mozambique worsened in the 1980s. Women have been victims of South African destabilization, suffering rape and violence as well as displacement from their homes. Their suffering has been compounded by an economic crisis that has impeded their ability to produce the family food supply. The increase in urban poverty caused by structural adjustment has been particularly hard on women. Adjustment must consider women's needs and capacities; the price of ignoring them is a deterioration in women's and children's health.

· 3 ·

Harvests of Disease

Women at Work on Zimbabwean Plantations

RENÉ LOEWENSON

TRAVELING ON A ROAD in a large-scale farming area in Zimbabwe, one commonly sees poorly dressed, thin women bending over huge plowed fields, weeding, planting, or harvesting. Many work with babies on their backs, entering the fields at sunrise and leaving after sunset. These are the women whose labor contributes to Zimbabwe's rich export harvests and southern African food security, while their own children experience some of the highest rates of malnutrition in the country.

The large-scale farm sector covers approximately 45 percent of Zimbabwe's land and employs 20 percent of its population. Through land expropriation, consolidated under the 1930 Land Apportionment Act and the 1967 Land Tenure Act, the large-scale farm sector secured the most favorable agroecological land areas. It received considerable state support through accessible credit, price subsidies, expenditure on infrastructure, and recruitment and control of labor (Clarke 1975; Duncan 1973; Riddell 1979; Stoneman 1981).

By the mid-1970s, foreign ownership dominated the sector; local farmers constituted 70 percent of producers but owned only 23 percent of land. In 1980, foreign multinational corporations such as Lonrho and Anglo American produced 75 percent of gross agricultural profits (Stoneman 1981). Relatively cheap credit and subsidized markets supported seasonal, labor-intensive crop production, which used fairly low levels of technology. Farmers made little attempt to diversify or to produce outside the natural growing season, and they met peak demands for labor by hiring seasonal workers, about two-thirds of them women (Clarke 1975).

Earnings in the sector were highly unequal: wages did not change in real terms between 1940 and 1970, and they decreased by 17 percent between 1963 and 1973 (Cross 1976). In 1965, 30 percent of agricultural income went to wages and salaries, declining to 23 percent in 1974. The share of profits rose from 23 to 32 percent in the same period (Riddell 1979), showing the pace of capital accumulation at the cost of declining workers' incomes.

To understand the specific role of women within large-scale farm production, it is useful to examine the conditions that women experience as members of the agricultural working class; their specific experience as female farmworkers; and recent changes in large-scale farm production in Zimbabwe to show how they have affected women workers.

General Conditions of Labor on Large-scale Farms

Living and working conditions on farms are generally worse than in other formal sectors of the economy (Du Toit 1977; Loewenson 1985; Loewenson 1986; Riddell 1981). Housing on private farm land is linked to employment; employers use the false assumption of temporary migrancy to justify the lack of workers' home ownership and improvements to housing. Although employers have made some environmental improvements for the diminishing core of permanent and semiskilled labor, the majority of unskilled workers have experienced little change since 1980 (Loewenson and Chinori 1986).

No existing laws define minimum living standards on farms. The lack of home ownership has defeated attempts to involve communities in making significant environmental improvements, which were possible after 1980 in areas in which urban inhabitants and peasants acquired their homes. On one farm, for example, workers resisted making bricks for toilets in their spare time: "We saw this to be unfair because this is not our land. When we leave this farm, we leave everything—hut and toilets" (Interview with permanent worker, February 1986, in Loewenson 1989). Emergent trade union structures have been unable to achieve their expressed goals of home ownership, legislated environmental standards, or significant environmental improvements (General Agricultural and Plantation Workers Union of Zimbabwe 1988).

Farmworker households struggle and often fail to meet their dietary needs. Despite the rise in real wages between 1980 and 1982, the total minimum wage of fifty Zimbabwe dollars was still 25 percent less than the estimated value of subsistence food needs (Loewenson, Zanza, and Mushayandebvu 1983). The ratio between wages and food needs has not improved since 1983 (Loewenson 1989). Large-scale farm areas have proportionally fewer commercial food outlets than peasant areas and almost no informal sector food markets (Loewenson 1985). Food prices are higher in farm stores than in urban areas (Chikanza et al. 1981; Loewenson 1984), and farm stores carry limited goods and their supplies are erratic. Most workers lack the time and inputs to supplement their food needs significantly through home production.

Illness in farm communities is a continuous feature of life. In a 1985 survey, 42 percent of adult women reported being ill within the past two weeks, the majority of illnesses being preventable, communicable diseases. Forty-three percent of children under the age of five years were reported to have had an episode of diarrhea in the past two weeks (Loewenson 1989). Malaria and sexually transmitted diseases were ranked as the most common adult illnesses reported to health services in large-scale farm areas, together with backache and traumatic injury (World Bank 1983).

Malnutrition is reportedly more common in farm labor than in other communities (Chikanza et al 1981; Loewenson 1986); 30 percent of children under five years old are chronically undernourished (stunted) and 16 percent are acutely undernourished (wasted) (Loewenson 1986). Although the 1981 and 1982 increases in real wages did not overcome the problem of below-subsistence wages, they appeared to reduce malnutrition among the children of farmworkers by 50 percent (Loewenson 1986). The most recent surveys carried out indicate, however, that since 1983 there has been little further gain in respect of stunting or wasting (Loewenson 1989).

Until 1980, health facilities were sparse, and their services were often limited to family planning and curative care. In December 1980, 75 percent of farmworker households in one survey did not have any contact with a health center and only 19 percent of children were immunized (Chikanza, Paxton, Loewenson, and Laing 1981). The provision of fixed clinics in large-scale farm areas has increased only marginally since 1980. Large-scale farm areas have over twice the number of people per facility as peasant areas, and the area covered by each health unit is seven times that of the peasant area average (World Bank 1983). Primary health care has expanded through increased coverage by mobile clinics and through the training of community-based farm health workers, who are the equivalent of community-based village health workers. Farm health workers are selected from farm labor communities on large-scale farms. Implemented since 1981, these primary health care programs face several problems: insecure tenure, weak organization, and the political isolation of workers, with nonpermanent women workers experiencing the greatest socioeconomic insecurity; a lack of worker representation on rural councils [1]; the absence of legislation stipulating minimum environmental standards; and an overall lack of fixed clinic facilities, support personnel, and state access to private land on which to build these services.

Households attempt to manage health problems themselves and avoid the costs of lost time at work and transport to facilities. In Mashonaland West Rural Council area in 1985, 30 percent of the households reported self-help as a first line of health care. Over half the surveyed households were using analgesics for minor illnesses, dosing themselves almost weekly (Loewenson 1985).

Occupational health has also received little attention, with negligible protective legislation, monitoring, or control of hazards, even though agricultural workers have among the highest levels of reported occupational accidents (Bwititi et al. 1987; Government of Zimbabwe Ministry of Health 1985).

Despite the legal amalgamation of peasant and large-scale farm area local government councils in 1988 under the Rural Districts Councils Act, farmworkers continue to be disenfranchised. Workers lack representation in local government, which marginalizes them from development planning. One farmworker said, "I wouldnt take our problems to the rural council because our interests are different from theirs. The council is interested in building roads, while we farmworkers are interested in improving conditions at work." (Interview with permanent farmworker, February 1986, in Loewenson 1989).

Agricultural workers were recognized as workers in industrial law only in 1980. Trade union organization is poorly developed, many farmworkers are illiterate, and farmworker communities are socially isolated and fragmented. These factors have undermined the workers' bargaining power and their sociopolitical development.

The Specific Impact on Women

Although poor conditions clearly affect the entire labor community, women carry an additional burden because they bear a large part of the social costs of production.

In the early colonial period, the withdrawal of male labor left women peasants to bear many of the costs of family subsistence and social well-being. The wage was oriented to meeting only the single worker's basic needs, leaving peasant production to support the rest of the family and future labor. Elderly, ill, or disabled workers were expected to return to peasant areas in which the lack of social services placed much of the burden of care on women. Capitalist production added to and transformed the precolonial exploitation of women, which was summarized by the late Samora Machel, president of Mozambique, (1973) in his comments to the conference of Mozambican women:

> To possess women is to possess workers, unpaid workers, workers whose entire labor power can be appropriated without resistance by the husband, who is lord and master. In an agrarian economy, marrying many women is a sure way of accumulating a great deal of wealth. The husband is assured of free labor which neither complains nor rebels against exploitation.

Women served as unpaid family labor within the peasant sector, and they subsidized the wage in the formal sector.

As land expropriation and capital starvation undermined peasant production, whole households became dependent on wage incomes. Families resettled on farms, mines, and in urban areas, and women continued to provide family subsistence and social welfare with even fewer resources. This penury pushed them into informal sector work, prostitution, or the worst jobs in the formal sector.

In the 1950's, large-scale farms increasingly employed women and children as cheap, seasonal labor. By 1970, one-quarter of the labor force was casual or seasonal, 65 percent of this casual or seasonal labor force was female (Clarke 1975). Employers in the sector met demands for labor in the planting and harvesting seasons by hiring the wives and children of permanent workers and additional casual workers of both sexes (Barker 1979). Men's employment was sometimes made conditional upon the employment of their wives. As a result, agriculture was one of the major formal sectors employing female labor; in 1985 agriculture accounted for 76 percent of formal women's employment (Central Statistical Office 1985; 1986).

As casual workers, women suffered the worst employment security and working conditions, with extremely low payment per unit of work (piece wages) and few employment benefits. Loewenson (1989) found that single or divorced women with no male wage earner in the household were particularly disadvantaged; their lives were a continuous search for work and the means to live outside sparse periods of employment.

A recent survey found nonpermanent women workers employed for up to six months of the year, working for up to twenty-one days a month in the peak period, and earning an average of 60 to 85 percent of the monthly minimum wage (Loewenson 1989). In periods of low employment, these women raised money through activities in the informal sector such as selling clothes, food, and mats, and through prostitution. Prostitution enabled some women to survive economically, although it clearly caused a great deal of social conflict within the labor community. One fieldworker reported in that survey, "Some casuals engage themselves with married men and if the wives discover this kind of connection, a rivalry emerges and results in fighting. I asked one lady how she felt in such an embarrassment and she replied, 'We can't help it; we love these men for the sake of help (money) and we can't survive without food for the children.'" (Loewenson 1989).

Employers use their perception that women and children are supplementary household wage earners to justify exploitative labor conditions. Nonpermanent women workers are deprived of rights accorded to other workers under the 1985 Labour Relations Act, such as leave, sick leave and gratuities, as well as ninety days of maternity leave. In practice, permanent women workers also often choose to forfeit this leave, unable to afford the 25 to 40 percent reduction in salary it implies. Working into advanced stages of pregnancy and soon after birth prejudices the health of both the women and their children.

Poor employment conditions, harsh living environments, and inadequate social facilities intensify women's dual burden of formal sector and domestic labor. Water collection, for example, is primarily a task of women and older children. When women are working all day, household water use is affected; less time can be spared for water collection, particularly given the communal nature of supplies and their relative inaccessibility. More sparing use of water raises the risk of water-related diseases, such as skin and eye infections and diarrhea. In the absence of adequate health services, women have to care for family members with these diseases.

Women and children are also responsible for foraging and for growing food for the household. These tasks and other activities such as food preparation compete with formal labor demands during peak periods. Attempts to meet both formal sector and domestic needs carry their own health risks. Meals prepared the previous evening or in the early morning and left standing for later consumption raise the likelihood of bacterial contamination (Loewenson 1989).

A year-long survey of the large-scale farm areas in 1985-86 found that women and children accounted for the highest proportion of illness reported by households; they suffered primarily from respiratory and gastrointestinal infections (Loewenson 1989). The major causes of maternal mortality on farms are reported to be septic abortion, complications of labor, obstruction in labor, postpartum and antepartum hemorrhage, puerperal sepsis, malaria, and sexually transmitted diseases—all products of poor access to care and of poor social conditions (World Bank 1983). In the 1985-1986 survey, the often female-headed households of nonpermanent workers also reported higher levels of child morbidity than the households of permanent workers. Child survival was lower, and death in the first year of life higher, in the households of nonpermanent than of permanent workers (Loewenson 1989).

Exposure to chemical, mechanical, and other hazards arises directly through work and through living in the work environment. The 1985-1986 survey revealed a seasonal dimension to such illnesses as gastrointestinal and respiratory tract infections. Peaks in illness coincided with peaks of employment, possibly reflecting the burden of work-related disease in adults and the effect of the withdrawal of women's labor from child care and other domestic activities. The demands of work commonly required women to leave young children in the care of older children, reducing maternal contact and making it difficult for mothers to respond to their children's health problems. As one woman contract worker commented, "When I go to work, the children remain at home alone...it is a problem to take the child to the field because he would cry and if I am to sit down and breastfeed him it would delay me in getting over with the day's work." (Interview with contract worker in Loewenson 1989)

In the absence of accessible curative care out of working hours, many women treated illnesses themselves with analgesics, tonics, and other commercial remedies, and they deferred seeking care until work was less intense. Nonpermanent workers held back from company health services for fear of losing employment and they tried to avoid being absent from work, fearing dismissal (Loewenson 1989). The time and wage costs to women workers of seeking medical care during periods of peak employment have undermined the use of health facilities, even when these are made more accessible. In a sample of mobile clinic visits on farms in the central Mashonaland area during a period of peak employment, a significantly lower proportion of households with nonpermanent workers than of those with permanent workers attended the clinic (Chi squared test, p<0.05) (Loewenson 1989). Significantly fewer children from the households of nonpermanent workers had health cards or were immunized (Loewenson 1989).

In the 1985-1986 longitudinal survey, although April, May, and June were the months of highest reported worker morbidity, the use of health facilities peaked only in the months of November and December. The April-to-June period was one of peak seasonal female employment and also one of higher earnings. Greater purchase of medications from stores and the use of private clinics nearer than free state facilities took place in these months in order to limit lost time at work. In the later part of the year, as cash demands for food, school fees, and other household requirements increased and as women's work decreased slightly, greater use was made of free state health care facilities (Loewenson 1989).

Female employment has thus emerged as a factor associated with ill health and depressed use of health care on large-scale farms. The association arises from the nature of women's employment and the lack of socially organized facilities to meet domestic needs.

Although formal sector work brings women out of the isolation and economic dependency of the home, the conditions of farm employment perpetuate their second-rate status and deprive them of any meaningful economic independence. Women's wages are well below poverty levels, and the almost constant demands of formal, informal, and domestic labor deprive women of the time for sociopolitical activity.

Employers justify the employment of women in repetitive manual work, such as cotton picking and harvesting of soya beans, by pointing to physical characteristics such as their "small and nimble fingers." The delicacy accorded in such descriptions belies the strenuous physical work inherent in these and other common tasks. Carrying forty-five pounds of water for over half a mile, bending for nine hours of weeding with a child on the back, or carrying irrigation pipes is hardly delicate work.

Oppressive social values add to the real economic insecurity of women to impede their effective sociopolitical participation. Loewenson (1989) found that women participated less than men in industrial relations structures such as workers committees. Although these are in theory open to both sexes and all types of labor, the poor social position of women, their insecure employment, and weak bargaining power as nonpermanent workers have combined to make their membership on workers' committees almost negligible. Women rarely have their own separate committees or are represented on the farm village committees, which are set up without legal or administrative power to solve family disputes (Loewenson 1989).

Women have therefore experienced the combined impact of the general conditions of social and economic poverty of large-scale farm labor; the poorest employment status, earnings, and working conditions; and responsibility for social and domestic welfare in the context of poor social provision of these services and overall poverty. Developments within the past decade have stimulated economic growth in the large-scale farm sector. Are they improving labor conditions? What has happened to the status of women workers?

Changes in the Large-scale Farm Sector in the Past Decade

From 1973, terms of trade for agricultural commodities declined, as crop prices fell on international markets and the costs of industrial inputs rose. Those units able to increase productivity through technological innovation and improved production practices were most likely to continue to reap profits, despite declining world prices. As a result, a number of trends have emerged in Zimbabwean large-scale farm production since the mid-1970s.

The use of machinery and chemicals resulted in more intense use of land and labor and reduced the proportion of land under cultivation. In 1978, of 39 million acres of large-scale farm land, only 1.5 million acres (or 4 percent of the total) were reported to be cultivated (Central Statistical Office 1988). In 1981-1982, only 10 percent of large-scale farms in Mashonaland were being cultivated and 18 percent of farms did not grow any crops at all (Weiner et al. 1985). In a regional assessment of large-scale farm use, Weiner et al. found that the most intensively cultivated districts, Bindura and Mazowe, produced crops on only about half of the available acreage. They concluded that one-half to two-thirds of Zimbabwe's prime land was being neither cropped nor fallowed (Weiner et al. 1985). Private control of this land area has meant that despite extreme land hunger in peasant areas and large numbers of unemployed rural workers, unused land has not been made available for production.

Industrial crop production such as cotton and coffee has expanded (Commercial Farmers Union 1986) with the use of greater mechanical, seed and chemical inputs. Chemical imports doubled in value between 1980 and 1982 (Government of Zimbabwe 1982), and the use of chemicals specifically allocated to agriculture rose by 333 percent from 1980 to 1986 (van Hoffen 1986). The use of fertilizers was 23 percent higher in 1985-1986 than in the previous season (van Hoffen 1986). The costs of fuel, chemicals, fertilizers, and irrigation rose by up to 400 percent in the six years following independence in 1980 (Commercial Farmers Union 1986; Government of Zimbabwe 1982; *Herald* November 4, 1985, 5), shifting profits upstream to their largely foreign providers.

Higher capital inputs and rising production costs increased farm indebtedness to private and state finance institutions (Clarke 1975; Riddell 1979). Between 1980 and 1985, Agricultural Finance

Corporation loans to the large-scale farm sector increased by 80 percent per loan, and the number of borrowers decreased from 2,500 to 2,000 (Loewenson and Chinori 1986). Local lending by private banks to agriculture increased from 60.9 million Zimbabwe dollars in 1979 to 112.6 million Zimbabwe dollars in 1986. In July 1985, Barclays Bank reported that in fifty randomly selected farm accounts, borrowings exceeded funds held by an average of 272,780 Zimbabwe dollars, and 10 percent of large-scale grain farmers lost their entire capital (Bernard Allen, chief lending executive of Barclays corporate lending division; Government of Zimbabwe 1986).

Increased use of mechanical, seed, and chemical inputs also led to more intense use of labor. Worker productivity rose by 50 percent in the decade prior to 1984 (van Hoffen 1986). Agricultural output increased, and the value of sales rose in 1985 to 47 percent more than in the same period in 1984 (*Sunday Mail* November 17, 1985, 2). Technological innovation and raised ratios of capital to labor have enhanced the growth of the sector.

Despite the rise in productivity, real agricultural wages did not increase. In addition, overall agricultural employment declined from the mid-1970s and by 1984, 100,000 jobs had been lost (van Hoffen 1986). There was also a shift to more nonpermanent forms of employment on a seasonal basis. In a 1985-1986 survey of large-scale farms, households with only nonpermanent workers constituted over one-third of the residents (Loewenson 1989). These households had lower levels of total employment (number of workers and days of work) than those with permanent workers; fluctuations in employment were primarily due to seasonal variations in women's employment (Loewenson 1989).

Employers have used nonpermanent employment to reduce the effect of progressive legislation adopted since independence. The 1980 Minimum Wages Act raised agricultural wages by 24 percent and gave leave, sick leave and gratuity benefits to permanent workers. With the passage of the 1981 Employment Act, which guaranteed employment security for permanent workers, employers rapidly reduced the number of permanent workers they employed and shifted to seasonal, contract, casual, and other nonpermanent forms of labor, often female (Zimbabwe Agricultural Workers

Union 1981). Employers viewed security of employment as "...
hindering the ability of management to maintain productivity."
(*Herald* August 10, 1987, 6)

Employers preferred to mechanize, supplementing a small core
of permanent workers with seasonal, nonpermanent labor.
Although agricultural development led to increases in output,
workers suffered from reduced employment and income. Surpluses
generated through increases in productivity were passed on through
high input costs and interest rates to the industrial and finance
sectors, much of which is foreign-owned. The process of concen-
trating capital in the agricultural sector generates increasing
proportions of underemployed and unemployed people, whose
material conditions and health appear to be significantly worse
than those of the fully employed. This economic trend particularly
affects women, given their poorer employment status and their
domestic burdens. The trend also undermines the collective
organization of labor, as unemployment, the shift to insecure
seasonal work, piece wages, and other forms of wage payments
related to output pit workers against each other in the competition
for scarce resources. This competition reduces labor's ability to
bargain collectively and to negotiate improvements in environmental and working conditions. Because there are few semiskilled or
permanent women workers, the trend to capital concentrations also
intensifies the social and economic marginalization of women who
work or seek work in the large-scale farm sector.

In other third world countries, rising unemployment is
associated with a growing national economic debt and declining
public sector budgets for social services, which undermine the
capacity of the state to meet social needs (Green 1986a; Green
1986b). One response to this problem in Zimbabwe's large-scale
farm sector is to meet the needs of permanent farm workers
selectively and to regard the seasonally employed and unemployed
as an invisible, surplus population (Jones 1986; Kemp 1986; Sircar,
Sajhau, Mavamukundau, and Sukanja 1985; Slesinger, Christenson,
and Caukley 1986). This surplus group has to rely on its own
resources and seek individual solutions for problems that are
essentially social in origin. Individual solutions place a large burden
on women, who have to implement them.

In the health sector, as the social provision of care becomes more inaccessible (whether due to real underprovision or raised opportunity costs), women individually take on the task of attempting to maintain family health. Certain approaches to health care reflect the view that health is an individual, often female responsibility, rather than a product of social and economic factors and actions. This view blames overpopulation on individual households for having too many children and targets women as key recipients of contraceptive programs. These programs may be implemented before the institution of more general forms of health care aimed at improving child survival. This view also attributes malnutrition to mothers' poor feeding practices and target these practices as the focus of nutrition education programs, without introducing corresponding action that would enable women to obtain the resources they need to implement the messages. This view places the blame for diseases arising from poor living environments on poor domestic hygiene practices, and tries to educate women to improve home hygiene.

This individual approach to health reinforces economic trends, which fragment the collective organization of labor. In the absence of social action on the underlying factors affecting health, women on farms bear the greater, more long-term individual struggle to maintain family well-being in the face of rising poverty.

These conditions demand sociopolitical action. In Zimbabwe, the trade union in the sector—the General Agricultural and Plantation Workers Union of Zimbabwe [2]—has initiated one form of this action. The union has begun a program of organizing and educating women workers. Its aim is to raise women's awareness and to strengthen general trade union organization by increasing membership and participation in this previously mar-ginalized section of the workforce. The union has consistently attacked harmful practices that affect women, such as piece wages and casual labor, and it has called for sociopolitical changes, such as home tenure in farm areas and worker representation in local government. The union recognizes that mobilization is an impor-tant task because the poor organization of women workers undermines working class unity as a whole.

As part of the social infrastructure on large-scale farms, the health sector also has a sociopolitical impact. The training of workers as farm health workers, the provision of primary health care, and community mobilization to make environmental improvements all raise awareness of the importance of social struggles in improving health. Health care providers have highlighted the lack of social organization as a factor limiting health actions (Government of Zimbabwe Ministry of Health 1985). Despite this, the health sector has been restrained in direct, strong support of worker organizations, particularly when such support engenders conflict with landowners.

There appears to be little space for compromise within the large-scale farm sector. The factors underlying disease are deeply rooted in the ownership and distribution of resources and profits, so that demands for improved health inevitably heighten conflicting class interests. The evidence of economic trends that worsen the socioeconomic status of labor in general and women in particular shows that family health is unattainable under current conditions of large-scale farm production, in which lives spent in strenuous labor reap harvests of poverty and disease.

· 4 ·

Nursing in South Africa

Black Women Workers Organize

NONCEBA LUBANGA

SOUTH AFRICAN black nurses' organized opposition to apartheid challenges a common stereotype of "apathetic" nurses. It is often argued that nurses see themselves as an elite profession, and that they are isolated from community struggles. As a result, they are unable to bring about change, despite their numerical advantage and potential power. Yet nurses, who are the largest group of health care providers, resist through hospital strikes, confrontations with authorities over patients' rights, and daily battles with the administrative hierarchy. Nurses occupy key positions in the health services, and without them, the delivery of most health care would not be possible.

A review of the struggles of black nurses enables one to focus on the black women who are the "unsung heroes" of the African struggle in South Africa. Black women have very little, if any, voice in the media, which seduce the public by promoting select personalities whose names fill the white press. The "little people" who are the backbone of an organization are forgotten. This chapter hopes to provide the African perspective on black nurses' struggles in South Africa. It draws upon interviews with nurses, the few published articles and unpublished papers on the subject, and on various historical documents.

Historical Overview of Black Nurses

African women worked initially as domestics in South Africa's growing cities because they encountered the least resistance from men and women of other racial groups in this kind of work and because, in the context of South Africa's racist society in which every white family aspires to have a servant, there was an ever-growing demand. In Johannesburg and other centers, the churches set up Native Girls Industrial Schools, in which girls were taught the rudiments of housekeeping. By the 1920s, female African domestic servants were becoming the norm in the Witwatersrand area and other urban centers.

African women with this rudimentary training could also work as domestics in hospitals and clinics. "Few African women had the educational qualifications to take the nursing certificate and many public authorities were reluctant to provide for the training of black nurses and believed they were not capable of passing the nursing examinations" (*Critical Health* 1988, 6). The first trained African nurse, Cecilia Makiwane, graduated from Victoria Hospital, Ciskei, in 1908; her statue now stands on the hospital's grounds. The Cecilia Makiwane Hospital in Mdantsane (East London), Ciskei, is named after her; so is the highly coveted prize, "The Cecilia Makiwane Medal of Honor," for the African nurse of the year.

Currently, 25 percent of South African women work outside the home. This level of economic activity is low compared with 50 percent of British women gainfully employed and 46 percent of French women. South African industry employs a few black women (4 percent of the African female population) in food processing, textiles, and clothing; this low-paid work is supposedly related to "women's domestic role," and women make up 83 percent of the blacks in this industrial workforce (Cock 1989, 7). The service sector (domestic service, catering, and laundering) accounts for 50 percent of black women workers (Jordan 1984, 10). Only 11 percent of African women find professional work, and 95 percent of professional women are teachers and nurses (Cock 1989, 7). African women are excluded from a wide range of jobs and are thus subject to double discrimination on the basis of skin color and sex (Luckhardt and Wall 1980, 311).

The South African Trained Nurses Association

In 1913, registered white nurses formed the voluntary and exclusive South African Trained Nurses Association (SATNA) (Searle 1965, 242). Its aims were to weld the nurses of South Africa into a united band of workers; encourage cooperation and take united action to protect the interests of the profession; encourage and maintain the highest ideals of nursing in South Africa; hold social and professional gatherings to discuss all matters affecting the interests of the profession; take steps towards the formation of benevolent funds or pension schemes; become more actively united through contact with similar nurses' organizations in other countries and with members of the profession throughout the world; take all possible steps to suppress the practice of nursing by unqualified women and to prevent abuse of the nurse's uniform (Searle 1965, 242).

These are noble aims for a profession like nursing but, strange to say, the African trained nurse could not be part of this association. From this one can see the shortsightedness of segregation and the tragedy of South Africa's racist policies. Kuper (1965, 217) observes that "Nursing bestows on an African woman new opportunities for freedom of individual development, but carries the burden of added responsibilities. It brings them past the threshold of Western knowledge, but shuts the door of equality in their faces."

Because of South Africa's racial policies, hospitals were segregated. In the late 1930s Afrikaner women's organizations demanded that the provincial authorities (which controlled most hospitals) should prohibit "European" nurses from caring for "Native" patients. They demanded that all hospitals admitting African patients should engage black nurses (Marks 1988, 8). Hospitals that admitted both black and white patients had separate wards for Europeans and for Africans. White nurses took care of white patients and black nurses attended to black patients. Only recently, because of an acute shortage of nurses, did black nurses begin to take care of white patients in white hospitals.

A few examples will demonstrate the segregated structure of South African health facilities. In the Cape Province, Victoria Hospital is a predominantly black hospital and only in very rare circumstances does it admit a white patient. Livingstone Hospital in Port Elizabeth is a hospital for Africans, so-called coloreds, and Asians; Provincial Hospital is Port Elizabeth's hospital for whites. Frere Hospital in East London has separate European and black sections for its patients. In Durban (Natal Province), Addington Hospital and King Edward Hospital are for whites and blacks respectively. In the Transvaal, Johannesburg General Hospital is for whites and Baragwanath Hospital is for blacks.

In June 1990, the government of F. W. de Klerk announced the end of segregation in health facilities. It remains to be seen how and to what extent this proclamation will be implemented.

Realizing that they could not belong to SATNA, the African nurses, led by a graduate nurse from Victoria Hospital at Lovedale, decided as early as the 1920s to form their own organization, the Bantu Nurses Association (BNA). In 1930 hospitals in and around Johannesburg were training African nurses, and the white matrons (directors of nursing) held a meeting to discuss the feasibility of forming an association like the BNA. Ruth Cowles (1933, 233), an American nurse and missionary, recalls how they decided it would be better to "lay emphasis upon the formation of Wayfarer [1] detachments than institute an association." The matrons thought that the Witwatersrand Branch should elect one of its (white) members to represent Bantu nurses. SATNA officials thwarted and stalled the African nurses' efforts to form their own organization until November 5, 1932, when they finally affiliated the BNA to their own association.

The BNA was more active than Borcherds (1958, 33) would have us believe. Nurses all over South Africa including one working in South West Africa (now Namibia) manifested great interest in the BNA (Cowles 1933, 233). The chief BNA aims were not very different from those of SATNA, except that the BNA also hoped to gain the confidence of the African people and be of great service to them. The BNA grew and by 1941 it had seven branches, a national headquarters, officers, and was holding national conferences (Wright 1985, 7).

Before continuing with the story of Black nurses, it is of interest to place the BNA in the context of some other South African professional associations, African trade unions, and African women's employment opportunities in the interwar period.

In the 1920s, Africans within the South African Teachers Association (SATA) found themselves in the same position as that of African nurses. African teachers broke away from SATA, a Cape Province organization whose membership comprised white, colored, and African teachers, because it did not adequately address their concerns. Africans felt that the problems they faced were different from those experienced by their white counterparts. The African teachers' grievances included a shortage of qualified teachers, too few schools, overcrowded classrooms, and inadequate equipment. At conferences, a separate committee debated these issues, which were always relegated to the end. Instead of talking about them in the open, SATA executives preferred to hold private discussions with officials from some of the predominantly African branches. African teachers referred to their position as "the kitchen department within SATA." In 1925 they formed the Cape African Teachers Association (CATA), and only a few branches in the North Western Cape remained in SATA.

Dockworkers founded the Industrial and Commercial Workers Union of Africa (ICU) at Cape Town in 1919; it soon developed into a general all-in union for non-European workers (Roux 1972, 153). The ICU gave birth in the early 1920s to the idea that the African worker is the creator of South Africa's wealth. This belief prevailed in the African community, and its acceptance marked the beginning of the political awareness that flowered in the 1930s and 1940s.

The Nursing Act of 1944

In the early 1940s, South Africa faced a severe nursing crisis. Contributing factors were bad living conditions, poor salaries, a shortage of nurses, restrictions on married nurses, and nurses leaving the profession (*Critical Health* 1988, 5). The withdrawal of 1,100 registered nurses from civilian services to staff military hospitals both locally and abroad during World War II also exacerbated the shortage of nurses. (As no African nurses were trained to occupy high-ranking posts, none was sent abroad at this time (Searle 1965, 258).) SATNA could not help nurses meet the crisis due to its undemocratic structure, aims, and objectives.

As a direct result of dissatisfaction with SATNA, white nurses started a movement in 1942 to form a new organization along trade union lines (Borcherds 158, 33). As Searle (1965, 248) notes,

This organization convened a meeting in the Red Cross Hall, Johannesburg, on 30th August, 1942, with a view to organizing the Nursing profession as a Trade Union ... the main speaker was a representative of the Garment Workers's Union. He stressed the fact that nurses were exploited by their employers (a statement which was unfortunately too true) and many of the long suffering nurses immediately reacted favorably to this sympathetic technique.

One or two radical medical practitioners spoke about the exploitation of student nurses, who were the main source of labor, but who received neither adequate salaries nor proper tuition.

In response to what became known as the "trade union crisis of 1942," the established leadership of SATNA and the Department of Public Health rapidly joined forces. Miss C. A. Nothard, then Matron-in-Chief of the South African Military Nursing Service, released Mrs. Sharley Cribb, the SATNA organizing secretary, to undertake a tour of all branches of the association and address mass meetings of nurses on the subject of trade unions. During these meetings, speakers warned nurses that the political aura associated with unions was contrary to the spirit of nursing (Searle 1965, 250).

What worried both the government and the SATNA leadership was the thought that nurses might "adopt a trade union mentality" and might even be persuaded to strike in order to improve their situation. Because of the possibility that Afrikaner nurses would branch off from SATNA and form their own separate association, and rumors that Afrikaner nationalists intended to make the reform of nursing a plank in their 1943 election platform, the government gave the Nursing Bill priority (Marks 1988; *Critical Health* 1988, 8). Trade unionists believed that if they had the nurses on their side, they would have the government where they wanted it, because "no government could withstand the political pressure which the withholding of nursing services would exert on them" (Searle 1965, 251).

SATNA campaigned vigorously for a closed shop professional association and its own governing body. All previous efforts had failed, but on this occasion SATNA was successful. The South African Nursing Act No. 45 of 1944, initially introduced to the House of Assembly as a private measure by Mrs. Margaret Ballinger, was taken over by the government and passed as a government measure (Borcherds 1958, 33). The South African Nursing Association (SANA) replaced SATNA as the professional association to which all registered nurses, student nurses, and midwives, irrespective of color, were now compelled to belong. (Under Section 38 of the Nursing Amendment Act No. 50, nurses of all categories who are practicing in South Africa are still required to be members, and failure to comply constitutes improper or disgraceful conduct, which is liable to penalties that range from a caution or a reprimand to the removal of the nurse's name from the register (Strauss 1981, 24-37).) SANA's objectives were to raise the status, maintain the integrity, and promote the interests of the South African nursing profession by making representation to government, provincial, and local authorities in regard to employment conditions, salaries, leave, and pensions (Searle 1965, 234). With the creation of SANA, the BNA was effectively eliminated.

According to *Critical Health* (1988, 8) "the non-racialism of 1944 Nursing Act seemed to represent a more liberal mood" than that prevailing at the creation of the segregated SATNA in 1913. Unity between nurses of different class, racial, and ethnic origins was a real, if superficial, possibility in 1944, given the liberal climate of the war years and the very small number of black trained nurses. Even at that time there were those who contested the achievements of the act.

SANA developed a highly bureaucratic structure that stifled progress within the organization. Nurses continued to express their discontent in the form of strikes despite the constraints laid down by SANA. Black nurses working at the Alexandra Clinic in Alexandra Township just outside Johannesburg went on strike in 1947. The clinic's board of managers claimed not to know what the grievances were. Ruth Cowles, who founded the clinic and worked there from 1926-1946, commented from the United States on the basis of news from her friends that the whole affair had resulted from intimidation by the "communists" who stirred up the community (Wright 1985, 9). What is surprising about Cowles' reaction to the nurses' strike is that she herself marvelled that nurses did not complain about the horrible working conditions, long working hours, and poor salaries. The Alexandra strike was a prelude to others.

The Victoria Hospital Strike of 1949

Victoria Hospital, Lovedale Institution, and Fort Hare form a triangle of educational campuses around the Tyhumie River in Alice, Ciskei (now one of the ten bantustans created by the South African government). Victoria Hospital was founded by James Stewart, head of Lovedale Institution, who recruited Dr. Neil MacVicar from Scotland as the first medical doctor. According to Phyllis P. Jordan (interview, May 7, 1989), who writes extensively about Xhosa history and culture, the training of African nurses for the whole of southern Africa started here. "It was an experiment which many in South Africa thought could never succeed, as Africans 'were not yet ready for such training and service.' But Dr. Neil MacVicar was visionary and the experiment proved a great success."

For many years Victoria Hospital trained colored and Indian as well as African nurses because no other schools were open to these women. Victoria, Lovedale, and later Fort Hare became the meeting places of black nurses and nursing students from all over South Africa and beyond. "A lot of good, dedicated nurses have come out of this hospital, nurses who have put their mark wherever they have been," notes Phyllis Jordan (interview, May 7, 1989).

In 1949, the student nurses at the hospital went on strike to protest the unfair dismissal of a nurse who had presented a petition of grievances to the hospital administration. One complaint concerned the composition of the hospital board: hospital authorities appointed two board members to represent the nurses. The nurses felt that they did not have a voice, that the appointed individuals represented not their interests but the interests of the hospital authorities.

Mrs. Jordan (interview, August 1, 1989), who was at Fort Hare during the strike, recalls:

> Going out on strike was a tough moral issue, for it involved withholding needed services to their patients. After a long debate on this question, the nurses decided to boycott the hospital and its facilities, but report for duty in the wards as scheduled. Even though a number of staff nurses were with the trainees in spirit, it was decided that they would not strike. Then the nurses walked out of the dormitories, the dining halls, and the classrooms. They camped on an open field just outside the hospital and went to the wards only on duty. This meant no beds, no blankets, no food, and no laundry services for them.
>
> When the communities around the hospital heard that the nurses were out on strike, they rallied round the strikers. Students at Fort Hare University, senior students at Lovedale, and some Lovedale teachers such as Mr. Mac Sipho Makhalima and the late Victor Hermanus brought mattresses, blankets, and groceries. Some wives of the African staff members at Fort Hare pitched in too with pots, pans, and food. The women from Ntselamanzi, Gqumashe, Dyhamala, and Gaga—the villages around

these campuses—came in to help with the cooking and the laundry.

Coordinating all these efforts were Mrs. Mzamane, wife of Professor Mzamane at Fort Hare, and Mrs. Xhaphile, wife of the Principal's secretary at Fort Hare. These women literally left their homes and children to attend to the needs of the striking nurses. From Lovedale came Tazana Mali and her sister Nonke Mali, a cook at Elukhanyisweni, Fort Hare. The laundry service organized by Mrs. Mzamane and Mrs. Xhaphile ran as smoothly as though there were no strike, and this was in the days when none of them had washing machines. Their resolve was that these nurses had to be clean everytime they went on duty, and they had to be fed.

The women did a marvellous job. Mac Sipho Makhalima kept up the nurses' spirits on cold nights, playing his piano accordion. Sometimes the people sang and he accompanied them, and sometimes they just listened to Mac playing.

A strong, active Youth League branch of the African National Congress existed at Fort Hare in those days. These young men not only assisted with material help, but also with getting legal advice for the strikers. Among the Fort Hare students were the late Robert Mangaliso Sobukhwe, president of the Pan African Congress of Azania, the late Nyathi Phokela, the late Themba Hleli, Ntsu Mokhehle, and others. One of the leaders of the striking nurses was Veronica Zodwa Mate (the present Mrs. Sobukhwe). Some people say it was the leadership qualities of this young woman that first drew Sobukhwe to her.

After two weeks of drawn-out struggle, with neither side prepared to back down, the nurses won. The hospital administration accepted their demands, one of which was that from then on whoever represented the nurses would be elected by them to the hospital board.

In his keynote address on behalf of the 1949 graduating class at Fort Hare College, Sobukhwe (1949, 7-8), who later served time in the notorious Robben Island prison, commented on the nurses' strike at Victoria Hospital:

> As you see for the first time since the practice was started, we do not have the nurses with us at this momentous night—Completers' Social. And the reason? The battle is on. To me the struggle at the Hospital is more than a question of "discipline." It is a struggle between Africa and Europe, between a twentieth century desire for self-realization and a feudal conception of authority.... The trouble at the Hospital, then, I say, should be viewed as part of a broad struggle and not as an isolated incident. I said last year that we should fight for freedom—for the right to call our souls our own—and we must pay the price.
>
> The nurses have paid the price. I am truly grieved that the careers of so many women should have been ruined in this fashion. But the price of freedom is blood, toil, and tears. This consolation I have, however, that Africa never forgets. And these martyrs of freedom, these young and budding women will be remembered and honoured when Africa comes into her own.

The story of the Victoria Hospital strike clearly shows how women display great courage when roused to action, courage that is often greater than that of men because women have immediate responsibility for children at home. It also demonstrates the solidarity that existed between nurses and the community and contradicts the notion that nurses are an elite group, totally isolated from their communities. Would the local people at Alice and the students and teachers at Fort Hare and Lovedale have rallied round isolated elites?

The Nursing Act of 1957

From the outset, black nurses faced discrimination. Despite their equal training, their salaries were far lower than those of their white counterparts. They had no access to the nurses' old age, convalescent, and holiday homes provided by the SANA and paid for out of nurses' dues (Marks 1988, 22; *Critical Health* 1988, 9).

From 1949, with the National Party in power, the government's object was to segregate the branches of SANA and remove the voting rights of the black nurses. In a referendum held in 1950, a small majority of SANA's members accepted the principle of racial segregation (Marks 1988, 25). Through the 1950s the composition of the statutory bodies, namely, the South African Nursing Council (SANC) and the SANA board, became steadily more favorable to the government's intentions. This shift was partly the result of government nominations to SANC and partly a reflection of the changed composition of the profession itself (*Critical Health* 1988, 9). (By the 1950s, 70 percent of the nurses were of Afrikaner origin, the result of recently urbanized and poorly educated Afrikaner women coming onto the labor market in the 1930s and 1940s and moving increasingly into nursing jobs (Marks 1988, 7).)

The Nursing Act of 1957 was a major turning point in the organization of nurses in South Africa, although it was gazetted merely as a consolidating measure and officially called the Nursing Amendment Act No. 69. As Charlotte Searle (1965, 234) points out, "all previous legislation relating to nurses and midwives had made no distinction on racial or other lines." The 1957 Act transformed this situation. Charlotte Searle, then the Director of Nursing in the Transvaal and already a dominant figure in SANA and SANC, was very explicit about the reasons. "She argued that 'non-European nurses' were only included on an equal basis in the 1944 Act because at that time there were very few of them and because the nurses were assured by the Provincial Authorities responsible for hospital services, that the authorities did not intend training black nurses for the full certificate" (*Critical Health* 1988, 9). According to Searle, (quoted in Marks 1988, 25),

> If we had known at the time that the policy of the provincial authorities was just the opposite we, and I for one, would certainly not have agreed to the introduction of the Bill as it was introduced in 1944. We would have fought

it to the last ditch. We certainly would not have liked to do something which would ultimately have wrecked the European nursing services in South Africa. At any event, because there was no problem at the time, it was decided that there would be no colour bar.

Margaret Resha, an African nurse who was in the opposition leadership, had this to say (personal communication, July 7, 1989):

In 1956, on hearing about the pending Bill which would amend the 1944 Nursing Act, to create separate registers along racial lines, African and European nurses around the Transvaal area had several meetings to discuss its merits. There were heated arguments between Black and White nurses. The White nurses tried to convince the Black nurses that apartheid was good for them and that since it was the country's new policy there was nothing wrong with creating separate registers in SANC and SANA. Realizing the futility of their pleas and of trying to reason with the White nurses, the African nurses decided to form the Rand Nurses Professional Club, which was later instrumental in creating the Federation of South African Nurses and Midwives (FOSANAM).

According to Marks (1988, 36), "The passage of the 1957 Nursing Act roused passionate opposition among black and a handful of white nurses. To add insult to injury, the state attempted to use the new registration forms to force the much-hated pass system on African nurses in order to use them as an example for other African women who were resisting the extension of the pass laws at the time."

This deception was very much resented by non-white nurses, particularly African women, because in order to obtain their identity numbers they had to report to officials of the Native Affairs Department, which was liable to issue reference books to them. They also objected to stating their race as "Native."

This is how Resha (personal communication, July 7, 1989) recalls the nurses' response to the threat of being used by the government for the extension of pass laws:

Between 1955 and 1956 many nurses joined the Women's League of the African National Congress (ANC) and the Federation of South African Women. The Nursing Council was instructed by the government to write to the matrons of the hospital requiring all the nurses to produce I.D. numbers. So, the Rand Nurses Professional Club elected me to go to the Native Affairs Department offices in Pretoria to inquire about the I.D. numbers. After being driven from pillar to post in these offices I finally landed a clerk who told me that the only way I would have an I.D. number would be for me to get a passbook.

The matrons, knowing the amount of resistance to carrying passbooks by women, never had the courage to tell the nurses that by asking the nurses to produce I.D. numbers for registration they meant passbooks. Realising that the hospital officials tried to trick them into getting the "passes," the nurses were seething with anger. They took the matter to the Federation of South African Women and Women's League of ANC and briefed them on the problems of the pass system and how it would interfere with their day-to-day work with their patients. Some of the problems they pointed out were: constant harassment by police and being searched for passes, which would result in lateness for work; absenteeism resulting from being arrested if one forgot to carry the pass on one's person; and disruption of their daily lives at home by constant police night raids making them psychologically and emotionally unfit to work effectively with their patients the following day.

The Federation of South African Women, the Women's League of ANC and the nurses organised a big demonstration of over 500 women and marched to Baragwanath Hospital, where they met with matrons and explained their reasons for resisting the proposed legislation. The matrons wrote back to the Nursing Council and the proposal was withdrawn for the time being. The next group of women to be victimized were the domestic workers, whose employers simply loaded them in their cars and then took them to the pass offices where they were issued passes.

Protest meetings took place at many hospitals. At a meeting of non-white nurses held during January 1958 at King Edward VIII Hospital in Durban, tempers rose to such an extent that the police were summoned, but the women had quieted down by the time they arrived. The hospital superintendent then announced that the Nursing Council had informed him that African women nurses who were not in possession of their identity numbers need not furnish them (Institute of Race Relations 1959, 179).

Non-white nurses at Johannesburg's Baragwanath Hospital also held protest meetings and announced that they would refuse to complete the forms. According to the *Star* (22 March 1958), the Federation of South African Women decided to arrange a demonstration in support of the nurses. The authorities feared that disturbances might result: the African townships were cordoned off from the hospital, roadblocks were set up, the police assembled in strength in the roads leading to the hospital, and it was reported that a ward had been cleared for possible casualties. As a result of the precautions taken, the policemen probably outnumbered the demonstrators who arrived at the hospital, the *Star* reported.

Resha continues:

In 1957 when the Nursing Bill was being debated in Parliament, nursing administrators and matrons were summoned to Cape Town to testify to the Select Committee that Africans were inferior and unsuitable to have the same nursing profession as whites. The African nurses who were still members of the same association with voting rights sent memoranda to the Select Committee expressing their opposition to the proposed legislation. They were ignored.

This led to the formation of the Federation of South African Nurses and Midwives (FOSANAM) which was launched in Johannesburg in 1957, even before the bill creating separate registers for nurses became an act. It was a protest organisation of predominantly black nurses and a few whites, with strong branches on the Reef, Cape Town, Alice, Transkei and other parts of the Eastern Cape Province. Nurses from Natal and the Orange Free State joined the federation at a later stage. With their slogan "Disease knows no colour," the nurses protested the introduction of segregation into their profession. They knew what had happened when the Bantu Education Act was introduced in 1954 and that the same was going to happen to their noble profession.

FOSANAM held its first conference in Cape Town in July/August 1958. A large delegation came from the Reef, among them Gladys Khala, the general secretary, Betty Nyama, the president, Mrs. Agnes Masina, Mrs. Greta Ncapayi. Mrs. Albertina Sisulu, even though a charter member of FOSANAM, did not attend the conference. Delegates came from the Transvaal and the Eastern Cape including Ciskei, Border, and the Transkei. The keynote speaker at the conference was Dr. A. C. Jordan, then a professor at the University of Cape Town. Using the Federation's slogan "Disease knows no colour" as the backbone of his address, Dr. Jordan exhorted the nurses to stand firm in their protest, remembering that they are the guardians of the health of the nation and that when on graduation they take the Florence Nightingale Pledge, they vowed that they would allow no power, no matter how strong, to stand between them and their service to the sick.

This first conference of some South African nurses promised a keen awakening to the issues of segregation facing the South African people and the awareness of a section of the educated elite who were supposedly the least socially conscious. The nurses took a political stand and defended their noble profession.

The government had anticipated opposition and, as in the case of Bantu education, had dangled sops all over and by stringent legislation made it well-nigh impossible for any nurse practicing and/or in training to follow her profession unless she was registered in the proper ethnic registers and in the case of Africans had a "Pass" or an I.D.

For the first time in the annals of the nursing profession in South Africa, African nurses were promoted to senior staff positions in almost all the clinics and hospitals that served an African clientele. A number of those promoted were the charter members of FOSANAM. The women had long deserved these promotions, for they were excellent health providers, their reputation beyond dispute. Co-opted now into the new structures, they were compromised and could not carry on their protests.

Contrary to what is written about how FOSANAM died in its infancy, Resha maintains that, in fact, the federation was quite strong for many years to come. It had branches all over South Africa and international support. The federation held its third conference in Orlando, Transvaal in 1961. "Unfortunately," as Resha complained earlier, "the media completely ignored coverage of these events."

An editorial comment in the *Lancet* (1957, 1182) highlighted the dangers and the implications of the 1957 Nursing Act. It also pointed out that, apart from its own leading article on the subject, there was virtually no coverage in the press. A circular to key members of the Royal College of Nursing and the National Council of Nurses mentioned the new act briefly. Whyte (1957, 786), writing in a British journal called *Nursing Times*, was the only reader to demand more information.

Victoria Hospital Nurses Strike, 1958

In March 1958 student nurses and some staff nurses and nursing supervisors went on strike to protest the expulsion of Sadie Stofile, a staff nurse who had allegedly attended a Youth League political meeting at Fort Hare College, Alice. The nurses demanded that the superintendent of the hospital, Dr. Cooper, give reasons for

Stofile's expulsion. According to Sikhumbuzo Maqhubela, a former Fort Hare student (personal communication, November 1989), Cooper's response was, "Even in Ghana they don't give reasons," a reference to Kwame Nkrumah's deportation of whites without explanation. Dr. Cooper ignored the students' demands and ordered them to go back to the wards. The students refused to work until their demands were met. They camped on the hospital grounds.

Once again the community rallied around them. A former Fort Hare student (personal communication, name withheld) recounts the following events:

As members of the Youth League of the ANC at Fort Hare and the student body, we gave support in the form of food and bedding. It was arranged with the kitchen staff that in the dining room, tables of ten would give up three shares of food per meal and tables of twelve would give up five shares. This amount of food remained in the kitchen kept warm until the students took it to Victoria Hospital grounds. The Fort Hare students were not permitted to enter the grounds, so transactions such as meetings, conversations, carrying messages, mailing letters, bringing in coffee, fruit, food, and sanitary pads were conducted over the fence.

The nurses dared not leave the premises of the hospital as they were told that re-entry would be denied. To give moral support and solidarity, some of the theology students would come and conduct prayers over the fence. The strike lasted a week and all of the nurses involved in the strike were dismissed. Most of these nurses, especially the registered nurses, were hounded throughout the country, their lives were shattered, some changed careers and others went to South-West Africa [Namibia].

With the support of the Fort Hare student body the nurses retained the firm of Mandela and Tambo to defend them. The firm instructed (the late) Advocate Duma Nokhwe to plead the defense case at Alice. The case was scheduled during the winter vacation (June/July). This was bad timing for the nurses; they needed the support of the Fort Hare students, who were on vacation. Their absence precluded the possibility of mass student demonstrations in front of the court.

Also, at this time there was a kind of euphoria around Alice because, for the first time ever, an African advocate was going to defend the nurses. There was a sense of pride in the community and also curiosity. Some people wanted to see "what an advocate looks like, what kind of a gown does he/she wear?"

The student nurses lost the case, but it was a political victory because it drew the attention of the public to the grievances that were expressed by the students, workers, and the masses around the country. However, the authorities were unrelenting, they held the stick end of the whip and with that they crushed the uprising with the hope that there will never be any more problems.

Nurses' Struggles from the 1960s to the 1980s

The nurses' struggle for improved working conditions and their protests against unjust policies within various health institutions continued unabated despite lack of support from official nursing organizations such as SANA. The alternative to SANA, in which membership is compulsory, would logically be a trade union. South African nurses were able to join unions that represented them as employees in certain situations; however, they were strongly discouraged from doing so (*Nursing News* 1983, 1).

The kind of intimidation to which union-minded nurses were subjected was demonstrated in the 1961 nurses' strike at King George Tuberculosis Hospital in Durban. According to Luckhardt and Wall (1980, 312-313), the strike was called to protest an incident in which Mrs. Malan, the matron of the nurses' residence, severely caned twelve nurses, allegedly for arriving in class a few minutes late. Skilled and unskilled hospital workers supported the nurses' demand for the expulsion of the matron.

With assistance from the local Hospital Workers Union, the nurses made several other demands. They wanted the policy of unequal eating facilities abolished. The African nurses were fed lower quality meals, were required to bring their own eating utensils, and they paid more than whites for their board and lodging. They also demanded raises in their scandalously low salaries. They demanded an extension of maternity leave to unmarried pregnant women to avoid fatal illegal abortions. They wanted an unemployment insurance fund. They demanded an end to the degrading practice that required African employees to make a cross when collecting their paychecks, instead of signing for them. And finally, they wanted African nurses to receive the same prophylactic treatment against tuberculosis that was given to all other employees (Luckhardt and Wall 1980, 312-313).

The nurses received support from local and international communities. Some of their demands were met, but the hospital superintendent refused to fire the matron. Twenty-two of the striking nurses were fired and all nurses were threatened with dismissal if they belonged to a union. Nursing authorities argued that trade unions could not act on behalf of nurses with regard to conditions of service or what professional acts the nurses might perform as these were the functions of SANA, the nursing association established by law (South African Nursing Association Constitution, October 1986). Yet it took a trade union to help nurses at King George Tuberculosis Hospital improve their working conditions.

In some countries, nurses engage in collective bargaining and are organized either in associations or trade unions to bargain collectively for better conditions of employment and nursing standards. The American Nursing Association (ANA) established an economic security program in 1946 that was designed to enable state and local associations to bargain for their members (Stern 1982, 9). In England, the Royal College of Nursing is the professional association that won certification as an independent trade union in 1977, and it is the collective bargaining body for nurses. British nurses are also represented by trade unions that are affiliated to the Trade Union Congress (Salvage 1985, 5). In Australia, the Royal Australian Nursing Federation is affiliated to the Australian council of trade unions and is the collective bargaining body for nurses (Gardner and McCoppin 1986). In South Africa, the 1978 Nursing Amendment Act (No. 50) made strike action by nurses a statutory offense with fines of up to 500 South African rand or one year in jail or both (*Nursing News* 1983, 1).

The 1978 Act provided for a nonracial nursing council to represent South African citizens; this provision effectively excluded many registered African nurses who, in terms of South African law, were citizens of "independent homelands." African nurses actively opposed forced segregation into separate "homeland" nursing associations, just as they opposed white nurses' domination of SANA (*Critical Health* 1988, 55, 56).

Despite the 1978 legislation, the 1980s brought many changes. Following the waves of trade union activism that began in 1973, hospital workers organized in Natal, the Transvaal, and the Cape. They joined such unions as the Black Health and Allied Workers Union, the General and Allied Workers Union, the National Education Health and Allied Workers Union, and the Baragwanath Health Workers Association. They aimed to break down barriers between different grades of health workers by bringing all hospital workers together in one organization, regardless of their skills and levels of training. These unions represented health workers in a wave of hospital strikes that began in the Transvaal with the action at Baragwanath, the "showcase" hospital in Soweto that serves a population of two million blacks.

Baragwanath Hospital Strike, 1985

In August 1985 *City Press* reported that sixteen nurses, picked from Baragwanath's "cream of the crop," were transferred to the Johannesburg General Hospital to take care of white patients. Hospital administrators took this move to ease the nursing shortage that threatened the white hospital's services. An investigation carried out by the Baragwanath Health Workers Association discovered that the nurses were not consulted prior to their transfer and that most of them were forced to go to Johannesburg. The *Star* alleged that skilled and experienced African nurses were being drawn from Baragwanath, which had a bed occupancy rate of over 100 percent, to nurse white patients in the Johannesburg hospital, which had a bed occupancy rate of under 50 percent (cited in *Critical Health* 1988, 59). The highly trained nurses were angry because felt that their skills were equally important for black patients who were already at a disadvantage. The Health Workers Association said it was "totally immoral and unacceptable" to use selected health personnel to upgrade the services of certain communities (*City Press* August 8, 1988).

In November 1985, hundreds of hospital cooks, porters, cleaners, nurses aides, messengers, and other auxiliary workers were arrested after downing tools to demand salary increases and better working conditions at Baragwanath Hospital (*Sowetan* November 14, 1985). Police arrested more than seven hundred men and women for attending an illegal meeting, which contravened Section 46(3) of the Internal Security Act of 1983, and for staging an illegal strike, which violated Section 65 of the Labour Relations Act No. 28 of 1956 (*City Press* November 15, 1985). Student nurses also went on strike against an 8:00 P.M. curfew, among other grievances, and, as they marched on the administration block, they were assaulted by hospital security guards wielding batons. Some injured nurses had to be treated at the emergency room.

The auxiliary staff and the student nurses had been brooding over their differences with the administration for some time and matters came to a head when the authorities were unable to meet their demands. According to the *Star* (November 11, 1985), a spokesman for the Health Workers Association said that hospital cleaners, messengers, porters, kitchen staff, and nurses aides had been agitating for pay increases for some time. Some of the workers with ten and twenty years of service were still viewed as temporary staff and others earned as little as one hundred and ten rand (U.S.$50) a month. Other grievances presented by the student nurses to hospital authorities were the poor quality of food, the victimization of student nurses who were outspoken, and the violent behavior of the Baragwanath Hospital security guards.

The *Star* (November 14, 1985) reported that by refusing to work, domestic workers and student nurses brought large parts of Baragwanath to a standstill. The hospital admitted no new patients other than emergency cases and transferred some patients to Leratong and to the Johannesburg hospitals. Operating rooms, several medical departments, and the kitchens closed down.

In a move that angered the black community even more than the hospital's refusal to consider the striking workers' demands, the authorities did not hesitate to dismiss seventeen hundred workers and student nurses. More than twelve hundred patients were left without adequate care until the South African Defense Force medical personnel took over many of the hospital's services, for example, nursing care, food distribution, and laundry. Even with this help, however, the hospital plunged into chaos, especially the emergency room. The laundry service was overloaded, wards were dirty, and food preparation and ward services were disrupted. The presence of soldiers in the wards performing nurses' duties was not appreciated by some nursing sisters. They felt that having soldiers around would have an adverse psychological effect on the patients (*Sowetan* November 19, 1985).

The striking workers and student nurses received support nationwide. Unions, various organizations, and fellow workers rallied to aid the workers dismissed from Baragwanath Hospital. Workers from several hospitals in the Johannesburg area, including Hillbrow, Coronation, and Natalspruit hospitals, demonstrated their solidarity with the dismissed workers. The United Democratic Front, the Azanian People's Organization, the Black Health and Allied Workers Union, and the General and Allied Workers Union all condemned the hospital authorities for dismissing the workers and refusing to negotiate with them. The Municipal and Allied Workers Union threatened to strike in solidarity if the grievances of the nurses and auxiliary workers were not met within a week. Some of the doctors, nurses, physiotherapists, and radiologists at Baragwanath Hospital sought a meeting with senior authorities to no avail. The medical staff threatened to strike, too, but deferred a final decision pending the outcome of the court action initiated by the dismissed nurses. The strikers were represented by the Health Workers Association and unions that had been organizing in hospitals, including the General and Allied Workers Union and the Black Health and Allied Workers Union of South Africa.

There was an outcry on the international front, and messages of support came from various professional organizations and institutions. Joseph N. Garba, the former chair of the United Nations Special Committee Against Apartheid, condemned the hospital's actions, saying the workers' stand once "again makes the public aware of the destructiveness of the apartheid system on social services in South Africa" (cited in *City Press* November 24, 1985). The American Public Health Association urged the United States Department of State to intervene to help bring an end to the abuse of health professionals, patients, and workers at Baragwanath Hospital. The ANA also pledged its solidarity.

SANA, which is supposed to represent nurses, condemned the nurses' actions in the whole affair. Recalling that nurses are prohibited by law from striking, SANA maintained that the student nurses had ruined their position within the nursing profession and that they had also damaged the public's trust in the profession. The association expressed dismay that the nurses sought union help instead of approaching SANA.

Three student nurses sought urgent court action to order hospital authorities to allow them to remain at the nurses' residence and to declare their dismissal unlawful. On November 25, 1985, the Supreme Court in Johannesburg ruled that the dismissal was invalid. Justice R. J. Goldstone ruled that the Transvaal Provincial Administration should reemploy the student nurses and auxiliary workers without loss of benefits. The *Star* (November 27, 1985) reported that the hospital reinstated all but one of the 940 nurses who had been dismissed and about 800 of the auxiliary workers who were fired for striking in support of pay increases.

The Transvaal Hospital Services lodged a complaint with the South African Nursing Council, alleging that the student nurses left their patients unattended during the strike. Because of the large numbers involved, the council selected eight nurses to appear before the disciplinary committee in Pretoria. The three complainants in the court application for withdrawal of the dismissal were among the eight who were summoned. The nursing council's punitive action came as a surprise to the nurses, who once again had to seek legal representation.

Hundreds of nurses from throughout South Africa came for the hearing, but they were locked out of the hall, which was packed almost three hours before the proceedings began. At the hearing, Mildred Makhaya, the principal matron of Baragwanath Hospital, maintained that, with the exception of student meetings, the nurses had no forum to air their views. They had felt increasingly inadequate in trying to communicate their grievances. Some had also been severely assaulted by other hospital employees (cited in the *Star* November 28, 1985). After desperate attempts to be heard by the authorities, the students had tried to approach Dr. Chris van der Heever, a senior hospital admission official. They waited three hours for a meeting, after he had twice previously refused to see them. The students' strike had not been premeditated; it was a spur-of-the-moment situation. The *Star* also reported that Mr. C. D. A. Loxton, a lawyer appearing for the nurses, said at the hearing that because of their special position in the community, nurses owed a duty to their patients; but because the Labour Relations Act did not allow nurses to strike, authorities had an added responsibility to provide mechanisms for the fair and proper airing of their grievances at all times.

In November 1988, SANA circulated to all its branches several proposed constitutional amendments that were to be debated in a constitutional congress planned for August 24, 1989. According to this document, "various changes and developments have made it necessary for the profession to consider further amendments to the constitution" (South African Nursing Association, 1988).

One such amendment concerns the status of nurses who are citizens of South Africa or territories that previously formed part of the republic. The new text would make nurses registered by the South African Nursing Council and practicing in the Republic of South Africa eligible for election to regional boards. The implication is that African nurses practicing in South Africa who are citizens of Transkei, Bophuthatswana, Venda, and Ciskei (the "independent homelands"), are South African citizens and therefore eligible for election to regional boards.

Another interesting feature of these proposed amendments is the elimination of any reference to race in the constitution. The reason given is that, from a professional perspective, the basis for association is common professional education and registration. The old argument that different population groups experience different problems in relation to certain issues such as conditions of service, no longer holds true. The implication of this proposal is that there will be a common voters' roll for the election of the eleven regional board members in the categories service, education, and private sector nursing.

The circular barely touches the reasons for SANA's change of heart. One can only speculate that it is no longer economical to exclude "homelands" nurses, given the acute nursing shortage in both black and white hospitals.

Conclusion

The role of African nurses in the economic well-being of the African community should not be underestimated. For generations nurses were the main source of economic viability for whole families. Student nurses were providers in the dual sense of providing the bulk of the nursing labor force and providing the family's income. Consequently nurses are always central to the African people's survival, and one can understand the strong support they receive from the community, which benefits from their training and their earnings. These nurses are hardly the "airheads" portrayed by Leo Kuper in *An African Bourgeoisie* (1965, 232) in which he talks of educated men who frequently commented that nurses were mainly interested in marriage and were politically unaware:

> They are only concerned with nail polish and status, and they come into contact with a certain amount of misery and want to help it but don't realize the political causes. They just go out with their boyfriends and come back to the same protected life. Their boyfriends don't speak politics with them, as it would just be a lecture. Their ambitions are shaped by the fashion and beauty columns which constitute their main literature. Smartness in appearance is what they desire above all.

It is unfortunate that the writer makes a blanket observation here about the lack of political awareness of the African nurse. Although one may agree with Kuper that nurses as a group rarely take a political stand, it must be pointed out that in the hospitals and in communities in which they work, they have been instrumental in initiating essential services to meet the needs of the people they serve. In large parts of the country, especially in rural areas, health care is in the hands of nurses. They plan campaigns and raise money to provide day care centers and nursery schools. They establish clinics in rural areas and women's clubs to teach nutrition; they encourage vegetable gardening and child health care. Nurses are saving many lives during the current wave of civil strife in South Africa. They treat victims of police shootings and hide them in their homes at the risk of losing their jobs.

It has been alleged that nurses rise up in protest only against poor working conditions and low salaries, but the question is, what workers do not? Political awareness does not develop in a vacuum. It has its roots in being aware of one's unacceptable condition and its reasons.

Nurses in South Africa play an important role in health care delivery. The African nurse, in particular, is an especially important link in areas where most doctors who are white do not speak the language or share the cultural background of the majority of patients who are black. The African nurses' contribution to black struggles has been enormous. They may not come out in great numbers in protest marches carrying banners, but by their day-to-day struggles within hospitals and communities, they are saving lives and making a significant contribution.

· 5 ·

The Health of Domestic Workers in South Africa

QUARRAISHA KHAN[1]

IT IS DARK OUTSIDE; a cold, gray, wintry morning. The silence in the shanty is suddenly broken by frantic movements. A blanket is hurriedly thrown off, a figure darts to a corner of the room, quickly washes her face and brushes her teeth, using the toothpaste sparingly. Nonkululeko makes a mental note to get more water from the water-seller this evening. She pulls on a few clothes and is ready to leave. As the door slams behind her, a mudpack falls off the wall of her temporary abode, which like the hundreds of shanties around it, was erected virtually overnight.

She reaches the bus-stop just as the bus arrives and fights her way onto the already overcrowded vehicle to get some standing room. The lucky ones around her who have seats are trying to make up for their interrupted sleep. As the bus winds through the township, picking up other passengers, she lets her mind wander to her children on the "farm." They are being looked after by her mother—are they all alright today? What if granny is sick? No! No! Don't let that thought go any further.

It's her stop. Several other women get off with her. As has become the custom, they walk together, singing or talking, protecting each other from being attacked by criminals that may be lurking in the area. It is a long walk to their places of employment, it really would be so convenient if they could use the half-empty buses reserved for whites that pass by every few minutes. Today, they all have to hurry because the bus ride had taken a little longer than usual. The "missus," as the employer is respectfully referred to, has already warned Nonkululeko about being late for work.

Nonkululeko reaches her employer's house, hurriedly changes into her work clothes, and starts in on her chores. First, the clothes have to be washed by hand and then put out to dry on the clothesline. The water is icy cold and her fingers begin to freeze. When the laundry is done, she begins to clean the inside of the house. The linen on the beds need to be changed, the rooms swept, the furniture dusted, and the floors scrubbed and polished.

The rumbling noises in her stomach remind her that in her haste this morning she had no breakfast. The bathrooms still need to be cleaned before it is time for lunch. After a quick meal, there is no rest, the ironing has to be done. She gets started with the ironing; there is more than usual this morning because of the guests staying over. When all of that is done, she has to help in the preparation of the evening meal.

At last! It is time to go home. Her feet ache terribly, the thought of the long walk ahead seems daunting. She still has to go home, buy some water, prepare her supper, and clean her shack. When will all of this ever end?

This is her routine from Monday to Saturday every week, every year. Sunday brings no more joy to her life—she has to use her salary prudently to buy her provisions for the week and ensure that there is enough money left over to send to the farm at the end of the month. Barely has she completed her chores before night falls. Too soon another week dawns, no different from the others before it.

Wait a minute! Tomorrow is the first Thursday of the month. This means that it is her turn to do the voluntary shift at the South

African Domestic Workers Union (SADWU) regional office. (The union has insufficient funds to employ more than one person per region and is dependent on members taking on tasks on a voluntary basis.)

Nonkululeko thinks back with joy on how she first became involved with SADWU. It was a day not so long ago when, utterly frustrated with her long, hard day at work and the realization that despite her sacrifices, the chances of her children having a life different from hers was remote, she joined a friend going to a SADWU meeting.

This meeting opened up a whole new world for her and filled her with hope. The experience of being with other women, all sharing a similar plight, who had come together to work collectively on protecting themselves, to devise strategies to improve their conditions of employment, and to challenge the authorities at every opportunity, made a dramatic change in her outlook on the future.

Nonkululeko's story is far from being fiction; any one of the thousands of domestic workers in South Africa could very easily replace Nonkululeko. This story is based on information obtained from personal interviews with several people, including domestic workers employed either as day workers or live-in workers, members of SADWU, concerned employers, and friends. It attempts to capture the ideas, feelings, and experiences of all those interviewed. (The choice of the name Nonkululeko is not arbitrary. It is a common Xhosa name meaning freedom. Its popularity reflects the extent to which this value is cherished.)

Domestic workers constitute a substantial proportion of the urban employed in South Africa. Health conditions of domestic workers are grossly under-researched, making it almost impossible to obtain accurate information on this hopelessly exploited labor force. One commonly known fact about domestic workers is that the majority are black women. Here, therefore, domestic workers are referred to in the feminine.

Domestic workers, together with farm laborers, belong to a unique sector in that they are not protected by government legislation relating to conditions of employment, for example, the number of hours worked, breaks during work, paid leave, sick benefits, minimum wages, and unemployment benefits.

Each employer determines the employment conditions of his or her domestic workers, which leads to wide variations with excellent salaries and benefits at one end of the spectrum, and almost slave-like conditions at the other end. This chapter focuses on the majority of domestic workers whose conditions of service lie somewhere between these two extremes. Despite occasional generalizations, it is important to bear these differences in mind and to be cognizant of exceptions.

The South African Domestic Workers Union (SADWU) was established in the late 1980s. SADWU, like other unions of domestic workers, must overcome the difficulty of implementing collective bargaining in domestic service. Traditionally, a single employer hires many workers, but in this situation, each worker has a different employer. Understandably, SADWU's negotiating power is still very limited, but it continues to grow.

Double Shift

Each day hundreds of women enter urban areas seeking employment; their only salable skill is their ability to do simple household chores. Their need for employment and fear of dismissal, which hangs over their heads like the sword of Damocles, both forces them to accept jobs with poor conditions of service and prevents them from negotiating better terms of employment. A triad of factors contributes to the oppression of domestic workers—racial oppression, economic exploitation, and sex discrimination.

The tasks of a domestic worker are demeaning, somewhat akin to modern day slavery. In a society where various racial groups have stereotyped roles, it is in keeping with existing norms and perceptions for domestic workers to be black. This tends to become a vicious cycle because the low status of domestic workers is used by racists to justify the continued subjugation of domestic workers in particular and blacks in general. Daily domestic servants work a double shift; they do household chores for financial remuneration first, and for their own house and family second. The fact that the majority of domestic workers are women follows social expectations that women do household chores. The demands of a chauvinist husband or boyfriend compound this stereotype: all day the domestic does the bidding of her employer and when she arrives home, her husband or boyfriend becomes her second boss.

Service benefits such as maternity leave, pensions, and medical insurance are rarely available to the domestic worker. Her low wages do not compensate her long working hours. In these inflationary times, she may take to theft as a last resort in order to supplement her meager income. If caught, her employer may dismiss her or have her arrested. This process of criminalization, besides having a major psychological impact on the domestic worker, is sometimes used by racists to justify their mistrust of blacks.

Some domestic workers live on the premises and their employers provide meals and accommodation. Live-in domestic workers may earn even less than their counterparts who commute from their own accommodation. The employers rationalize that they are providing the domestic worker's essential needs and the servant therefore has little need of money. The low wages paid to live-in domestics is not seen as a salary but as pocket money for her incidental expenses.

Domestic workers, like most other black workers, confront a dire shortage of accommodation when they enter urban areas to seek work. South African laws are not designed to make their attempts to find employment or accommodation easy. Formerly, the availability of accommodation at the employer's residence was an important consideration for women choosing domestic work. The reality is, however, that this accommodation often comprises small, poorly ventilated rooms with little privacy. Accepting the accommodation also means being at the beck and call of the employer at all hours and adhering to the employer's rules, which are especially harsh with regard to visitors.

Currently, many domestic workers choose to live in squatter camps. In these precarious surroundings, they attempt to create some semblance of a family life and to feel that they are part of a community. There are particular hardships associated with this choice; the most important is that of insecurity of land tenure. A domestic worker leaves the squatter camp every morning hoping that her shack will still be there when she returns in the evening.

Like many townships, squatter camps have no electricity, lack water-borne sewage, and have no piped water. Domestic workers have to explore other sources of energy; several are expensive and strain their already limited budgets. In addition, the alternative energy sources increase the hazard of fire.

Water assumes the value of liquid gold and obtaining it involves spending time in long lines at the water-seller or communal tap. Because storage facilities are inadequate, it is difficult to maintain the sterility of water. Limited financial resources necessitate the sparing use of the water and lead to the development of unsanitary conditions.

Transport is another major problem because the domestic worker usually lives far from her place of employment. She spends many hours every day traveling to and from work. Buses are generally overcrowded, infrequent, and expensive. Workers are known to spend up to 30 percent of their wages on transportation.

To reach the bus-stop from their homes, domestic workers use unlit, eroded pathways as roads. Walking in the gloomy light of early morning when their day begins, and back home in the early evening on their return, is quite hazardous. The perils are particularly pronounced after a few days of rain, which increases dramatically their chances of slipping and injuring themselves.

The domestic worker faces the daily threat of being robbed or raped. She often takes short-cuts to get from the bus-stop to her employer's house. She must constantly be on the lookout for thieves or rapists who may be lurking in these areas, especially on payday.

The term "girl" is often used to refer to a domestic worker, even though she may well be forty years old or even a grandmother. This way of referring to a domestic worker continues even in households that have employed the domestic worker for many years. "Girl" sums up the the way the employer views a domestic worker. It implies that the domestic worker is incapable of making her own decisions and it denies her status as an adult.

The domestic worker is further belittled when she is insulted by her employer's children. Sometimes, they even assault her, although many of them were nurtured in their infancy by the same domestic worker. The children observe their parents' interaction with the domestic worker, and they view their abuse of her as an acceptable form of behavior.[2]

Stress

Many domestic workers share large amounts of time with their employers, particularly if the employer is a housewife. During the long hours spent together, a domestic's employer constantly hovers over her, supervising the execution of duties. This stressful relationship, together with the physical demands of the position, has a substantial impact on her mental health.

Her complete immersion in work, at both her employer's and her own house, leaves the domestic worker with little time for recreation or relaxation with her family. She finds herself unable to spend time with friends or to participate in community activities.

The immense stress and anxiety experienced by the domestic worker arises from her numerous problems—job insecurity, the demeaning nature of her job, poverty, concerns about the health of her children, and her lack of rest and recreation. These may manifest as physical ailments, for example, headaches, depression, and hypertension.

The domestic worker's long day is followed by the work of caring for her own family. By bedtime she is physically exhausted. She has little time for herself and often neglects her own health. She fears taking sick leave because it may mean losing her job. As a result she often appears at a hospital when the disease process is so severely advanced that recovery is likely to be protracted.

"Washerwoman's Hands"

Domestic workers are at higher risk of certain occupational health problems. Their work is labor intensive; washing clothes by hand

and scrubbing and polishing floors are but a few examples. Many employers possess labor-saving devices such as washing-machines, dishwashers, and floor polishers. They keep these machines in reserve, however, to be used by the employer in times of crisis, such as when the domestic worker has not come to work.

In the course of their daily work, domestic workers use harsh detergents and cleaning agents, rarely with any protection such as gloves. "Washerwoman's hands," the result of damaged fingernails and nailbeds from constant exposure to highly abrasive cleaning agents, is rampant among domestic workers.

There are two clinical presentations of "washerwoman's hands." The first, paronychia, is a condition that results from the destruction of the cuticles following inflammation caused by bacterial infections. The fingernail becomes thick and distorted. This damage can lead to a more severe condition, onycholysis, which is the separation of the nail from its underlying bed. The second presentation is "housewife's dermatitis," which results from prolonged exposure to strong alkaline soap powders and detergents. Other causes of this condition include allergies to various household cleaning agents and working with certain foods. "Housewife's dermatitis" can cause the complete destruction of the nail (onycholysis, described above). It is an extremely painful condition that requires treatment with antibiotics. The recommended treatment includes the use of gloves, a pair of cotton gloves under rubber gloves. Healing is prolonged and can take up to one month.

The many hours spent kneeling to scrub and polish floors is associated with arthragia and arthritis, which are common among domestic workers. Some domestic workers experience respiratory allergies as a result of breathing the fumes of insecticides or the ammonia of cleaning agents.

The Absent Parent

The following scenario reflects the uniquely insecure lives that blacks are forced to lead in South Africa. Thandi grew up in a rural area and had her first child when she was still in school. The baby's father, also a student, went to the city to look for a job and never returned. Her second child's father is a mineworker in the Transvaal and, for most of the year, he lives in a men's hostel, which excludes wives and children. Thandi and the children saw him once a year and occasionally received some financial support from him. Thandi eventually went to work as a daily domestic, leaving her children behind on the farm in her ailing mother's care. She shares a temporary abode with her current boyfriend whom she met in the city. He has a wife and family in a rural area and sees them once a year. Ironically, being together and offering each other comfort has created a far greater measure of stability and consistency than anything else in their lives.

The apartheid system, together with the lingering effects of the now abolished influx control and migrant labor system, systematically eroded the concept of the family unit and conjugal stability among South African blacks. Economic necessity forced mothers to abandon their attempts at subsistence farming and to enter the labor market in urban areas. They left their children behind on farms that were little more than houses in dry rural slums. The children were cared for by other family members, who were generally much older and not in the best of health themselves.

The lucky domestic worker is able to see her family twice a year; she spends the rest of the time agonizing over their well-being. Her children grow up with little parental support or guidance. The absence of parents, not unexpectedly, leads to poor school attendance and performance.

The Road Ahead

Now the question is, "How does one begin to address these problems?" The mainstay of the solution to these problems lies in legislated protection of the domestic worker's rights and a change in the attitudes of South African society to blacks, women and workers. But these are long term aims. Current attempts to improve the lot of domestic workers are largely directed through SADWU. Its growing membership bears testimony to the need for a legal avenue for domestic workers to channel their grievances.

Encouraging employers and employees to enter into written agreements that stipulate the period of employment, salary, working hours, paid leave, benefits, and transport costs is one of SADWU's major campaigns. During August 1989, SADWU took this campaign one step further by organizing several marches to government offices; workers demonstrated and presented lists of their demands to officials.

This campaign is but one attempt to focus attention on the plight of domestic workers. The ultimate solution lies with a government that respects the concept of a family unit, conjugal stability, the right to adequate housing, and access to medical care. It requires the abolition of the apartheid laws and the creation of legislation designed to protect the domestic worker by enforcing a minimum wage, providing benefits such as maternity leave, workers' compensation, medical insurance, a pension scheme, the right to collective bargaining, and the protection of workers from exploitation and discrimination.

Ultimately, the rights of domestic workers will best be protected when blacks have access to government-level decision-making processes. This may only be feasible, however, when the bigger political battles are won and all South Africans, regardless of race, sex, or creed, have equal rights in a non-racial democratic South Africa.

· 6 ·

Women, Work, and Nutrition in Nigeria

SABA MEBRAHTU

RESEARCH ON WOMEN in development is split into studies of women's work, which emphasize women's productive functions, and reports on women's nutrition, which focus on reproduction. The split is unfortunate because women's work affects women's nutrition in several ways. The time women devote to agricultural and household chores determines the amount of energy expended and therefore the amount of food needed to supply that energy. In subsistence production, the time devoted to farming and food processing may also determine the amount of food there is to eat. The hours thus occupied also determine the time available to seek health care or to prevent infections. Disease prevention is important to nutrition because illness saps the energy required for work, and because some common infections such as diarrhea interfere with food absorption. The narrow focus of health studies on reproduction is regrettable because nutrition affects other aspects of women's well-being.

The critical decisions that affect women's work and nutrition are taken within the household. It is unfortunate that both bodies of literature ignore this dimension of women's work and nutrition. The household, here defined as the compound of the husband's extended family in which a man, his wife or wives, children, and other relatives all live, mediates the allocation of resources, including labor, time, and food. Women's workload, the quantity and quality of the food women eat, and the frequency and type of health care they receive vary with the political atmosphere and economic circumstances of the household.

Studies that take the household as their focus tend to use simple operational definitions and to isolate each of its functions, for example, production, consumption, dwelling, and decision-making. In practice, these functions overlap within households and many transactions, such as exchanges of labor, money, and gifts, occur between households. Ethnographic observations of behavior within and between households need to be highly perceptive and analytical, if they are to capture the household and community factors that are important to rural women's nutritional welfare.

Women do more than men to achieve household food security and nutritional well-being, particularly in rural areas. Women also carry more responsibility for weaning infants, who are nutritionally the most vulnerable population. Because women's roles in developing countries cut across several disciplines—agriculture, economics, sociology, health, and nutrition—there is a need to use a multi-disciplinary, holistic, and analytical approach to research on women's work and nutrition.

The aim of this study is to develop a new conceptual framework for the analysis of women's work and nutrition. It is important to consider women's nutrition, not only from a biological perspective, but also from a political and economic perspective. The study takes for granted that women have special nutrition needs and are most vulnerable during childbearing, pregnancy, and lactation. But women are also disadvantaged in terms of their socioeconomic and political position in the household, community, region, and nation.

The chapter is based on ethnographic fieldwork on the intermediate mechanisms affecting women's nutrition. The factors considered are social and demographic characteristics; household interactions; the demands of farm work on women's labor, time, and energy; food consumption; and efforts to prevent infectious diseases, which interact synergistically with nutrition. The ethnography involved participant observation and open-ended interviews with forty-four women. The fieldwork was carried out in 1987 in three Yoruba villages with a combined population of 2,150 in Kwara state, western Nigeria. Laduba, Budu Agun, and Ago are a cluster of agricultural villages that are located eighteen miles from Ilorin, a major urban center, to which they are linked by an excellent road and bus service. Islam is the predominant religion and Yoruba the main language. Fifteen percent of the population is originally Fulani. For detailed historical accounts of Yoruba and Fulani power politics and population settlement patterns see Sudarkasa (1973) and Fadipe (1970). This study is preliminary, and a more quantitative and definitive investigation should follow it.

The chapter begins with a review of the status of our knowledge of women's work and nutrition. We next consider decision-making and resource allocation in the household, in an attempt to localize women's power. This section includes a discussion of the importance of mutual support networks and women's participation in community organizations. We then describe women's work in trading, farming, and housekeeping in some detail, and we analyze the impact of women's workloads on time and energy expenditure. There is also a brief discussion of women's perception of their work and workloads. The final section summarizes women's health and nutritional status.

The Interrelations between Women's Work and Nutrition

Important contributions to the broad field of women's work include methodological studies that evaluate household labor, which is unpaid, and work in the informal sector, which is not accounted for in national statistics (Beneria 1982; Goldschmidt-Clermont 1982, 1983, 1984, 1987). A second group of studies analyzes the patterns of time that women allocate to their many tasks (Acharya and Bennet 1983; Berio 1984; FAO 1983; McSweeney 1979; Mueller 1979; Spiro 1980a; UN 1987; White 1984). A third area is women's significant contribution to agriculture and the multiplicity of their work roles (Adeyokunnu 1981; Ay and Nweke 1984; Boserup 1970; FAO 1979, 1987; Longhurst 1982; Okeyo 1979; Spiro, 1985, 1980b).

The case for the importance of women's labor contribution to agriculture and of women's multiple work roles is now well established (Adeyokunnu 1981; FAO 1987). Of course, the value of the work varies widely, depending on women's socioeconomic status, whether they live in an urban or a rural setting, etc. Available data indicate that, particularly in sub-Saharan Africa, women spend more time doing paid and unpaid work than men do. This comparison holds across most socioeconomic categories (Adeyokunnu 1981; FAO 1987; White 1984). Ester Boserup's (1970) classic work on women's role in economic development revealed that women do 70 percent of the agricultural work in Africa. The United Nations estimates that women accomplish 70 percent of food crop production, 100 percent of food processing, 50 percent of animal husbandry, and 60 percent of marketing (Longe 1985; Olawoye 1985).

Despite this evidence of women's productive activity, most medical and nutritional studies of women's nutrition focus on women's reproductive functions. Maternal and child health programs focus on the child rather than the mother, and they generally treat maternal nutrition as a function of child welfare and nutrition. As Hofvander (1983, 9) notes, maternal nutrition "focuses attention on women as mothers, on their nutritional status as it relates to the bearing and nurturing of children." One cannot deny the importance of these issues for women and children in developing countries; the point here is that research on women's health is imbalanced because it emphasizes women's reproductive functions over their productive functions (Eide and Steady, 1980).

Some recent studies focus on women's need to balance their productive and reproductive tasks; this often involves a trade-off between time spent caring for children and time allocated to cultivation, marketing, and housekeeping (Engle 1981; Joekes 1987; Leslie 1987; Nieves 1981). Unfortunately, these studies make no attempt to link women's productive and reproductive work responsibilities to their nutritional welfare.

Conceptual and empirical research that addresses women's overall nutrition in terms of their economic activity is scanty. In the words of Hamilton, Popkin, and Spicer (1984, 27), "anthropologic, economic, and sociological studies on women have rarely considered women's nutritional status to be a unique area of study." Exceptions to the rule, a few studies link seasonal patterns in women's workload to women's nutrition (Carp 1983; Chambers 1983; Chambers, Longhurst, Bradely, and Feachman 1979). These authors, however, do not take account of the politics and economics of the households within which women function; that is, they do not consider seriously the role of the household in decision-making and the allocation of labor and other resources.

The complex dynamics within rural households have yet to be explored and examined. A few authors attempt to take account of household factors in the design of research and policy strategies (Acharya and Bennet 1983; Fapohunda 1988; Guyer 1986, 1988; Imam 1988; Jones 1986; Rogers 1983). These studies challenge the simplistic assumptions of the economic model that treats the household as a utility maximizing, joint decision-making unit.

Decision-making and Resource Allocation in the Household

The measurement of decision-making powers poses serious problems. Gathering information on sensitive issues of family interaction is complicated; individual reports of decision-making processes are not precise; and various participants may offer differing accounts of events or be unwilling to admit the true distribution of influence. Rogers (1983) argues that one should bypass decision-making processes and accept instead the observation that household resources are allocated on the basis of the perceived economic contribution of household members. To avoid these methodological problems, Acharya and Bennet (1982) used an innovative survey instrument, which attempts to capture the interactive process. They found that women's participation in decision-making increases with their economic contribution to the household and that their involvement in subsistence agriculture affects participation negatively.

Evidence on the extent of Yoruba women's participation in household decision-making is conflicting. Some authors (Adeyokunnu 1981; Sudarkasa 1973) indicate that women defer to men. Our study shows that women play a considerable role but that decision-making powers are divided along gender lines. Men generally determine crop production and their wives are in charge of marketing and domestic activities. Men also have considerable say in decisions on child health care, such as where to take a child for treatment (to a traditional healer or a biomedical clinic). Also, other people play important roles in household decision-making processes; they include the head of the compound, the compound's wives organization whose leader is generally the eldest wife in the compound, and other members of the extended family. The frequency of these people's involvement in routine decisions may not be as great as that of members of the nuclear family.

According to our ethnographic observations, the allocation of authority varies by socioeconomic status and area of decision-making. Socioeconomic factors that affect women's input in decision-making are their contribution to the household cash economy, marital rank (senior, second, or youngest wife), number of children, proximity to family and kin, and household and community perceptions of their status and their work. In general, because trading is women's domain, women dominate market decisions; however, if a husband sponsors his wife by giving her financial assistance to set up trading, he will play an important role in decision-making. A majority of the Yoruba interviewed said that farming was men's domain and that men took decisions in this area.

Resource Allocation

If one is unable to measure decision-making powers directly, one can deduce women's influence by examining their access to resources. There is ample anecdotal and some definitive evidence indicating that household members have unequal access to goods and services such as land, labor (their own and other household members'), cash income, food, and health care (Ay and Nweke 1984; Fapohunda 1988; and Rogers 1983). Empirical evidence on household members' differential access to land is limited. Although there is an increasing trend towards rural landlessness and forced movements of households to ecologically marginal land in much of sub-Saharan Africa (World Bank 1981 cited in Allison 1985; Cashman 1986), the mechanisms behind land scarcity in the African region have not yet been subjected to rigorous scrutiny Allison (1985).

There is no landless class in our study villages, but access to "good" land is an important issue, particularly for women. In general, the area is moderately suitable for the cultivation of yam, cassava, sorghum, maize, sweet potatoes, tobacco, millet, cotton, cowpeas, soybeans, groundnuts, cashew nuts, and some fruit. Annual rainfall varies between 1,200 and 1,300 millimeters. Women acquire land from their husbands and generally it is not "good" land. Men borrow or inherit land. About half of the male farmers could borrow land from community members for a minimal fee; the rest inherited land from their forefathers.

Access to Income

The fact that households do not pool income is now well documented (Fapohunda 1988; Guyer 1988, 1986; Rogers 1983). Women appear to have more access to the income that they earn than to that earned by their husbands or other household members (Loose, 1980). There is conflicting evidence on male and female spending patterns.

In rural Yoruba households women and men keep separate accounts and have different obligations to the household economy. Men provide staples, health care, and in some instances children's school fees; women provide soup ingredients, clothing for themselves and their children, baby foods (some fathers buy infant formula as a status symbol), school supplies such as books, and uniforms, and sometimes school fees. The important question is how often and under what conditions these obligations are met.

There seems to be no simple or single answer. In the study population, the acquisition of food and nonfood items varied according to the woman's income, parity, and marital position.

Access to Food and Health Care

There does not seem to be the pronounced gender difference in the distribution of food in African households that is reported for south Asia, perhaps because African women have a well-defined and explicit economic role (Guyer 1980 cited in Rogers 1983). It was extremely difficult to make any systematic and meaningful observations. Generally, everyone ate from a common dish, but clearly adult males took precedence; the patterns were not as clear among young males and females.

Women had minimal access to biomedical health care. They could not visit a doctor or nurse without their husband's consent. The population relied for most preventive and curative health care on a relatively well organized group of traditional herbalists and midwives. The nearest biomedical health care was at Gommo, about six miles from the study villages. Very few people visited the hospital. When they did it was mostly for serious or severe conditions. The low rate of biomedical health care use is most probably due to the high costs of transporation and prescribed drugs (there were no visiting fees) and to the time required to travel, to wait to see a doctor, and to obtain drugs.

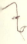

In conclusion, women's power to make decisions that affect the household, particularly the allocation of key resources, is limited. Husbands control the allocation of land and access to biomedical health care. Men also in effect determine the allocation of labor, which is the rural household's scarcest resource, by confining their contribution to certain tasks and designating others as "women's work." In the areas of income and food, the evidence is less clearcut. Women have less access than men to income, especially to money earned by other household members; and adult men appear to claim priority in the distribution of food within the household.

The Work Women Do

Traditionally in Nigeria, men farm and women trade (Fadipe 1970; Marshall 1964; Sudarkasa 1973). Women are also responsible for all household activities such as cleaning, food processing, carrying water and firewood, meal preparation, and child care and feeding. Recent findings suggest that the traditional sexual division of labor is changing; women are playing more active roles in farming (Adeyokunnu 1981; Cashman 1986; Spiro 1980b, 1985). In our study, we observed a considerable overlap in gender task allocation. Some women farm in their own right (up to 30 percent), and the rest work on their husbands' farms. Women indicate that they are increasingly being forced to farm more and to shift from yam to cassava. Most men (up to 95 percent) assist their wives in the arduous task of processing cassava. Both men and women participate in trading, although "women know the market better." Children assist in all household activities including farming, food processing, and household chores.

Trade and the Market

The market also plays a dominant role in people's lives: extensive economic tansactions and social interactions take place during the periodic markets held every five days. Women are central to the marketing system, and virtually all women engage in trading at some point in their lives.

The importance of Yoruba women in marketing is undisputed (Cashman 1986; Fadipe 1970; Sudarkasa 1973). Forty-one of the forty-four women we interviewed claim that their primary occupation is trading. The woman designated "mother of the market" has an influential political position in regulating internal market mechanisms. The crops traded are yam, maize, sorghum, cassava, melon, shea nuts, locust beans, some groundnuts, and a few vegetables. Imported nonfood and food items, such as cigarettes and canned milk, are also sold. Women engage in both short- and long-distance trading. Short-distance trading takes place within or around the village; long-distance trading takes place in nearby major urban centers and may entail a five- to ten-day round-trip. Most of the women (35) trade in the villages; only six travel to market their goods. Generally, the women sell processed (21), cooked (10), or raw (7) food; a few (5) sell nonfood commodities.

Trading requires a high initial capital investment, which is an obstacle for the many women who have limited access to credit and limited savings. A number of women in our study population believe that the initial investment pays off and gives a better return on their labor than farming does.

Urban middlemen are now replacing rural women traders who lack sufficient transport, storage facilities, and capital (Cashman 1986; Mebrahtu 1989). Their competition may reduce women's contribution to the urban and rural economies, particularly in the sale of mass produced goods and the long-distance trading of raw food products.

Women Farmers

Farming is the main source of Yoruba livelihood. Traditionally, farmers used a mixed cropping system known as intercropping, which is an adaptation to ecological and socioeconomic factors such as the distribution of rainfall, labor requirements, returns to land and labor, and the need to minimize risk. They practiced organic manuring, bush fallowing, and long fallow periods, and they used low levels of technology and little capital investment. These traditional farm practices are undergoing a major transformation. Increasing population pressure on land causes farmers to shorten fallow periods, replace organic manure with chemical fertilizers, and use tractors to plow (IITA 1988; Longhurst 1984). Maize and cassava are replacing yam and sorghum (Dheil 1982; Nweke and Winch 1980). As Steiner (1982) points out, the relatively new competing crops are easy to cultivate, store, and transport. The women I interviewed confirmed these advantages: "cassava is becoming more important because it is easier to grow and store, and we rely on it when yam is finished before the harvest season."

There is conflicting evidence on the degree to which women participate in farming. Cashman (1986) and Spiro (1985) document a steady increase in the number of women who farm in their own right and an increase in the acreage cultivated by women between 1976 and 1985. The contradictions may reflect changes over time or evidence from different parts of the country; for example, Longhurst (1982) studied northern Nigeria whereas Adeyokunnu (1979) made a national survey. There are also important differences between remote villages and rural areas that are near major urban centers. In remote villages, relatively more women farm, plant the same crops as men, and have equal rights or at least easier access to land (Ay and Nweke 1984).

Interestingly, thirty-eight of the forty-four women interviewed said that they prefer trading to farming. They explain the shift to farming as a measure necessary to the household's survival, which is jeopardized by economic and demographic pressures. The major reasons they give for the pressures are that the availability of family farm labor has declined over the years as men emigrate from the villages; that population pressure reduces family and household access to "good" land; and that their husband's farm income no longer meets the household's needs for food and money because of inflation and rising prices. The women's response to these pressures is to increase their farm work and to adopt a different mix of crops.

Although not as closely studied, another important factor in changing cropping patterns is male migration to urban areas for employment. Increasing rates of migration from rural to urban areas are well documented in sub-Saharan Africa (Diehl 1982). Yam is primarily a man's crop and when women take over men's production responsibilities, they substitute women's crops such as cassava and maize. The division of crops into men's and women's is very common in the western region of Nigeria and in the eastern part of the country (Nweke and Winch 1980). Women's crops include cassava, cocoyam, maize, and a wide variety of vegetables. Yam, a highly revered food crop, is strongly believed to be a man's crop. The Yoruba regard it as the "king of foods," and a special crop "from the ancestors." Men make all production, marketing, and consumption decisions on yam. Women make similar decisions on cassava, maize, and vegetables when they do not interfere with yam (Nweke and Winch 1980).

Another reason for growing cassava is the increased demand for processed cassava, *garri* (fermented, dried, shredded, and fried cassava granules), and *lafun* (fermented, dried, and ground cassava flour). Women are involved in processing and marketing, as well as growing cassava, which makes this operation economically viable.

Farm Labor Demand, Crop-Mixture, and Nutrition

Shifts in traditional cropping patterns should be carefully monitored for their possible impact on household food security and nutrition. For women, who experience serious constraints on their time and energy, a good crop mixture is crucial. Preferred is one that does not require too much labor, time, or energy, that can meet the household's needs for adequate food, and that has a potential for generating income. For these reasons, cassava is women's choice. As Longhurst (1985, 10) says: "farmers, in the way they choose crop mixes, planting time and the range of cultivation methods and factors, have in mind their own rationale for household security." But unless it is intercropped with legumes, cassava has adverse effects on child nutrition in poor households because its protein content and energy density are limited (IITA, 1988). Whenever infant weaning foods are nutritionally deficient, agricultural development projects should consider this eventuality (Brown et al., 1988).

Unfortunately, there is no evidence to link cropping patterns to women's nutrition; thus far all of the research has emphasized child nutrition. As Cliff notes in Chapter Two, however, when children are malnourished, women (who provide their food) also suffer nutritional deficiencies. Women in our study villages, especially those who farm in their own right, perceive the demands of time, labor, and energy to be relatively high in farming. The majority (38) feel that it is much better to trade than to farm. Many of the women (25) are concerned about their health as a result of the heavier work of farming. In the women's words, farming "consumes a lot of energy...women age faster ... they do not feel good ... and their stomach turns upside down." Their reluctance to increase their farm responsibilities is understandable.

Housework

Women's contribution to the well-being of their households is clear and obvious. Their responsibilities include the supply of fuel and water, virtually all food processing and food preparation, and housecleaning. Children help their mothers in housework and husbands help in processing cassava (soaking and drying are generally done near the farms). Women are also responsible for the care of children, the elderly, and the ill.

In these tasks women receive important social support from community organizations, members of the compound, cowives, and other relatives. Unfortunately, not many investigations of women's work and child feeding practices take account of this assistance (Buvinic, Graeff, and Leslie 1987; Engle 1981; Joekes 1987). Indigenous community organizations are common and important for women and men in the villages studied. They represent untapped resources of leadership, knowledge, and means of communication (Howes and Chambers 1979; Mebrahtu 1989). By coordinating efforts among individuals and households, they enhance and strengthen ties between households and increase economic efficiency and benefits.

We identified at least twenty-eight local organizations, each with a different purpose, agenda, and goals. Members generally pay a nominal membership fee and attend all meetings. A man may be a member of a women's organization by contributing money for which he receives social and economic benefits, but he cannot attend meetings; the same is true of women in men's organizations. There are three functional categories of organizations: specialized occupational organizations of self-employed, commodity-specific producers and traders of agricultural and nonagricultural commodities, and other wage-labor occupations (bricklayers, vehicle owners and drivers, hunters, herbalists, etc.); small credit organizations with rotating funds for short-term loans; and social, ceremonial, or religious organizations.

Women in our study population have access to and participate in a wide array of indigenous organizations, which are usually more accessible to poor women than are the well-established international, government, and private health agencies. The small, nonbureaucratic structure and mostly female staff give these agencies a distinct advantage in dealing with women's economic and health issues. Established health institutions could probably capitalize on the expertise and information that women's indigenous organizations can offer (ICRW 1989).

In the three villages under study, social and community support in childcare is important for mothers with toddlers. Infants are almost always carried on the mother's back, even when she is working, "until the baby is too heavy," usually at eighteen months. Although women receive labor support from the community during the busy seasons, the responsibility remains theirs. Thirty-nine of the women interviewed said they alone are responsible for preparing food for their husband and children; the other women rotate this chore among cowives, mothers, and mothers-in-law who live in the same compound. Thirty-three women said that, generally, they alone do most of the housecleaning; the others receive assistance from mothers, daughters, mothers-in-law, and co-wives.

Women's Workload and Nutrition

Unfortunately, women's work is generally evaluated in terms of its duration rather than physical intensity, which gives only a partial measure of fatigue and physical suffering. There are ways to estimate individual energy requirements on the basis of basal metabolic rates and of time spent on activities involving different energy costs, but they are relatively imprecise and indirect (Longhurst 1984; Lunven 1983).

Labor time is the rural household's scarcest resource. Time allocation data are limited for the African region, but it is clear that women have very little free time. In Burkina Faso, Mossi women have only eighty free minutes in the first fourteen waking hours (McSweeney 1979), in Botswana women have 20 percent less leisure time than men (Mueller, 1979), and in Nigeria women have only four hours of leisure time per week (Spiro 1980a).

There are methodological issues in collecting time use data. Differences exist between recalled and observed time use; recall is usually inaccurate, and observation is expensive and highly intrusive. The general recommendation is to use random spot observations (White, 1984) with a small sample of time duration observations (Rogers, 1983). Another problem with time use data is that productivity differs significantly between individuals, which confounds evaluation of time used for a given task. The best available method derives imputed value of time from the market price of household produced goods (Goldschmidt-Clermont 1983). This evaluation is not of concern here because we examine women's time use in relation to energy expenditure.

In general, there is more speculative than definitive evidence on the links between women's workload (energy expenditure) and women's nutritional status (energy intake and infections) (Eide and Steady 1980). Some secondary information has been obtained for male workers in Nigeria (Longhurst 1984) but there is none for women workers. In Burkina Faso, female farmers have a mean energy expenditure of 42.2 Kcal/Kg (kilocalories per kilogram of body weight) in the dry season and 52.6 Kcal/Kg during the rainy season (Blieberg, Brun, and Goihman 1980); male farmers in the same region expended 40.2 Kcal/Kg during the dry season and 57.7 Kcal/Kg in the rainy season (Brun, Bleiberg, and Goihman 1981). During the peak agricultural season, men's workday (17.3 hours) is longer than women's (3.7 hours), but during the dry season men rest more than women. On average, women work more than men year-round (Hamilton, Popkin, and Spicer 1984).

Women's perception of their work conditions and workload is critical to any meaningful framework for the analysis of nutrition. Many of the women (36) in our study villages claim that they are "contented" with their primary occupation which for the majority (41) is trading. About half (17) of those who claimed that they were satisfied also said they saw no alternative, because they lacked money and skills for other work; we may say they were "passively contented." The other women gave a range of reasons for being satisfied with their occupation: relatively high profit margins (11), work keeps one busy (3), meets home consumption food needs and enhances purchasing power (2), easy work (2), and access to a new technology and skill (1). These women could be called "actively contented." Seven women stated that they were not happy with their work because of low profit margins, saw no alternatives, and were "actively discontented."

Yoruba women perceive trading to be highly compatible with their other responsibilities as mothers and wives. The majority of women traders (41) do not feel that they are either overworked or too busy. Twenty-one indicated that they have ample time to rest, and six stated that their work is easy or could be carried out in close proximity to their homes; fourteen declined to give any reason.

We speculate that over the years, Yoruba women for whom trading is a primary occupation have adapted their work to the cultural, political, and economic context of their households, that their work is responsive to household economic needs and family obligations such as childcare, and that it also fits their physiological needs. Women recognize their need for adequate rest. The trend to increasing demands for women's labor in agriculture may, however, upset this balance. Women recognize that farming rerquires more energy than trading does.

Conclusions

The division of research into the two major areas of productive work and "reproductive" nutrition without considering the political and economic atmosphere of the household within which women operate has important policy implications. Development programs concerned with women's welfare treat women "as passive beneficiaries of the development process" (Longwe 1985). Longwe urges a shift from "a mere concern with women's welfare towards a programme for women's increased empowerment." She argues that, despite resistance from male dominated government bureaucracies, it is necessary to put women on an equal footing with men in the decision-making process, and that women's participation is the most important element in development planning.

Women's health needs to be recognized as an integral part of both productive and reproductive household functions. To address the reproductive bias in women's health and nutrition research, policymakers and researchers should take into account women's roles as economic producers. Poor women in rural areas work more and have more responsibilities within the household than men. Although, women's central position in the agricultural economy is now widely recognized, particularly in sub-Saharan Africa, it has not been seriously considered in agricultural research and development efforts, in part because conventional measures of economic activity underestimate the magnitude of women's productive roles and fail to acknowledge the value of unpaid work outside the formal sector.

A holistic and integrated approach is necessary to address fully women's issues in agricultural production, marketing, food processing, storage, preparation, and consumption, especially infant feeding practices. These issues should be studied from political and economic perspectives before an intervention program is launched. Emphasis should be placed on strenghening women's economic survival strategies and their indigenous political and economic organizations.

The case of Yoruba women in Kwara state is an interesting one. Women experience economic and demographic changes such as male migration from rural areas and declining real income as pressures at the household level. These pressures affect the type and amount of work they do. Women are farming more than before and trading less. They are planting cassava because cassava demands less labor, time, and energy and gives higher returns to labor and land than yam. More research is needed on the implications of this shift in cropping patterns and women's increased involvement in agriculture.

In conclusion, future research and development programs on women's health and nutrition should take a broad perspective incorporating political, economic, behavioral, agricultural, and biomedical issues (ICRW 1989). Important research priorities are the economic and demographic trends that will continue to have direct and indirect effects on women; in sub-Saharan Africa, these include high population growth rates, agricultural intensification, technological innovation, urbanization, and a growing proportion of households headed by women, which augur increases in their workloads.

· 7 ·

Gender and Health in Africa

MEREDETH TURSHEN

AT A PARIS family planning clinic, a request to see Mrs. B was answered with a sad shake of the head. Against her will, Mrs. B had been sent back to Mali because, without her husband's permission, she had asked the gynecologist for "breathing space between pregnancies." At twenty-five, she already had four children and complained of constant fatigue. Mr. B accused the gynecologist of being a bad doctor because there was no baby that year. He took his wife to a private obstetrician, who ordered a sonogram. Mrs. B begged the staff not to reveal her secret, but a new technician, unaware of the compact, gleefully pointed out the intrauterine device to Mr. B. Within two weeks, Mrs. B was divorced and dispatched to Bamako.

Women all over the world pay a price for the symbolic "room of one's own." They struggle to hold onto their personal and professional identities in the face of family pressures to marry, to have children, to advance a husband's career, or to sacrifice their own. The price seems to be keyed to social power—the lower the woman's status, the higher the price exacted. There is a lot of controversy and confusion about the social power and status of African women. Are they independent, self-supporting, and largely autonomous, or are they subordinate to men? Does their status as cultivators and traders with a separate income earn them respect and freedom from male domination, or are they triply exploited— working the equivalent of one job in their husband's enterprise, another in domestic chores, and a third on their own account? Have their economic contributions to their households bought them social and political equality or merely added to their responsibilities without commensurate increases in authority? These are crucial questions for women's health, which in the first instance is determined by women's ability to control their productive and reproductive labor.

Reproductive Labor

There are multiple definitions of reproduction. Edholm, Harris, and Young (1977) disinguish three aspects: biological reproduction, reproduction of the labor force, and reproduction of the social relations of production. All three affect women's health. In all three cases, the questions asked here are, who is in control, how is that control maintained, and how do women respond or resist?

Women everywhere pay with their lives for their lack of control over biological reproduction, but the rates at which they pay are strikingly different in industrial and underdeveloped countries. African maternal mortality rates are 2,000 per 100,000 live births in Ethiopia, 1,680 per 100,000 in Benin and 1,500 in Nigeria; these rates, which are the world's highest, refer only to deaths in hospitals and medical institutions. (One can gain an idea of the proportion of deaths these rates represent by considering the percentage of births attended by health staff— 58 in Ethiopia and

34 in Benin; no figure is available for Nigeria). Maternal mortality rates in industrial countries are 13 per 100,000 live births in France and 2 per 100,000 in Canada (UNICEF 1989, 106-107; World Bank 1989, 226-227). Unsafe, illegal abortions may be responsible for half of the maternal deaths in underdeveloped countries. Hidden in the extraordinary African figures is the price women pay for male control of their productive as well as their reproductive labor.

Who controls biological reproduction? Stichter and Parpart (1988, 10-11) state correctly, "By and large the regulation of reproduction has been through male-dominated social institutions of marriage and kinship.... The struggle over how many children to produce and who shall have rights to them is the content of the 'class struggle' in the reproductive realm." Vock (1988, 83) questions the flat feminist assertion that men control women's fertility: "Fertility may be, however, one area where males cannot successfully exercise complete domination." Vock is right; the evidence is complex. The case of Mrs. B suggests that women resist, more or less successfully, and that they pay a heavy price when they fail.

Chaulet and Ladjali (in Ladjali, Chapter Eight) describe an unwritten, unspoken marriage contract to bear a certain number of children: Algerian women must produce four or five children, including one or two sons, before contraception can be contemplated. Even after this contract is fulfilled, not all couples agree to limit the size of their family, and complicated negotiations may ensue between husbands and wives and other members of the extended family. Chaulet and Ladjali ascribe women's reluctance to use contraception to the lack of alternatives to motherhood for social prestige and status.

The degree to which society influences these household decisions is sharply underlined by recent data on Algerian women in France. The numbers of children born to Algerian women in France have declined spectacularly from 8.92 in 1968 to 4.24 in 1985 (*Le Monde* June 27, 1990, 24). The assumption is that in France, women have access to education and subsequently to vocations and careers, in other words to a social status that is not defined solely by marriage and motherhood, and that the alternatives prompt them to take advantage of birth control to limit family size. This may be true of the second generation, but it is less clear that foreign-born wives of migrants find more freedom in France. The natality data may reflect the fact that their husbands, wholly dependent upon wages (which may not have been the case in Algeria) and aware of both the risks of unemployment and the high costs of child rearing, decide that four or five children are enough. This decision to stop may bring no change to the wife's status.

Is an alternative social status sufficient to give women the power to wrest control of their fertility from men? New social values have changed family models among Senegalese immigrants in France. Fainzang and Journet (1988, 151) say of polygamous households in Paris that female authority no longer rests with the senior wife—in chronological order of marriage—or the wife who has the most children, but with the one who arrived first in France or the one who has the highest level of education. Polygynous households present special circumstances regarding reproductive control and seem to obey Stichter and Parpart's (1988, 10-11) stricture that the male-dominated social institution of marriage regulates reproduction. Fainzang and Journet (1988, 92-97) say that rivalries between and among co-wives extend to competition in reproduction. When one co-wife is pregnant, a second also tries to conceive, in order to retain her place in the household.

A good example of wives' difficulty in negotiating the terms of sexual relations is the new problem of using condoms as protection against AIDS. Schoepf et al. (this volume) describe Zairian wives' inability to persuade their husbands to use condoms, even after "consciousness-raising exercises in empowerment." Condoms require men's cooperation at the time of intercourse in a way that modern contraceptives such as the Pill and the intrauterine device do not. When using condoms, women lose control of contraception, which passes back into men's hands; for a woman to impose the use of a condom requires a more equal balance of power in the couple.

AIDS has brought issues of African sexuality to the fore. Although the causative virus can be transmitted through blood transfusions, contaminated medical instruments, and from mother to fetus, it is sexual transmission that has drawn the attention of the media, researchers, and the general public. Some reports claim that African sexuality favors the heterosexual transmission of HIV because promiscuity and prostitution are widespread. The World Health Organization has made dire predictions about the impact of this new, fatal, communicable disease on African society. Because at least half of the cases occur in women, an understanding of sexuality is important to African women's health.

Sexuality

African sexual permissiveness, it is said, begins soon after the initiation rites of puberty for girls and boys and continues after marriage for wives and husbands; Caldwell, Caldwell, and Quiggin (1989, 3-4) state that its basis is a societal model characterized by (inter alia) "The emotional and economic weakness of the conjugal bond [which] is reinforced by polygyny, the great age gap between spouses, and the long postpartum period of sexual abstinence." They also attribute importance to the social segregation of men and women, which, they say, makes extramarital relations easier for both women and men. They claim that this is a radically different pattern of behavior, which amounts to "an alternative civilization."

One should note in general that Caldwell, an eminent Africanist demographer, and his coauthors are comparing African sexual *practice* to the *ideals* of the Judaeo-Christian tradition (which they call the Eurasian model), not to the historical record of actual European or North American sexual behavior. They read the (English-language) anthropological studies of African societies out of the historical context of the transatlantic slave trade, a century of colonial domination, and recent economic exploitation. They pay little attention to the biases of the mostly male, mainly white, collectors of the data, although Victorian notions of sexuality probably influenced many Anglo-Saxon scholars. Finally, they tend to give equal weight to ethnographies from the 1920s and the 1980s, despite enormous changes over the past sixty years. Their statement about the emotional weakness of the conjugal bond must be examined in detail.

Divorce, Infidelity, and Intimacy

Divorce and infidelity are Caldwell, Caldwell, and Quiggin's measures of the emotional weakness of the conjugal bond; intimacy is a third measure examined here. Caldwell, Caldwell, and Quiggin (1989, 12) assert that in sub-Saharan Africa, divorce and separation are frequent. Given the North American experience of divorced women falling into poverty, high rates of divorce are an important issue for African women's health. Caldwell, Caldwell, and Quiggin attribute marital instability to the emotional and economic weakness of the conjugal bond. They do not quantify frequency and do not say whether men or women initiate divorce. In some traditional societies, when men controlled divorce procedures, there were few divorces (see Parpart 1988, 117, on changes in early colonial Zambia). This is one reason divorce may not be a good indicator of marital instability. Another is that polygyny, far from encouraging men to divorce, legitimizes a second relationship while preserving the marriage. Women are deterred from seeking divorce because it means leaving their children, who belong to their father. Also, divorce rates are keyed to social and economic conditions and may rise in periods of instability associated with rapid change. Rates are therefore historically specific.

It is difficult to quantify the frequency of divorce in Africa because not all marriages are registered. Kaufmann, Lesthaeghe, and Meekers (1988, 222-223), in a study of data from the 1960s and 1970s for six African countries [1], estimate that 17 percent of women married before the age of twenty will be divorced before the age of thirty-nine. The rates in France, a predominantly Catholic country not known for high rates of divorce, are the same: 17 percent of marriages celebrated in 1970 ended in divorce by 1987 (INSEE 1990, 298). If marital instability is common in Africa, it seems unrelated to any specific "African civilization."

Caldwell, Caldwell, and Quiggin think that, although infidelity is common, it is not a cause of divorce. It seems to me impossible to determine whether African men are more frequently unfaithful to their wives than are European men, let alone which group suffers more guilt as a result. It is clear that when men exercise power over women, women experience a good deal of sexual harassment, as Schoepf et al. report for Zaire in Chapter Eleven.

The double standard appears to be global, and it probably accounts for both men's marital infidelity and premarital sexual adventures. I find it hard to believe that African bachelors have a monopoly on "sowing wild oats," but Caldwell, Caldwell, and Quiggin (1989, 13-14) say, "men frequently do not marry until their late twenties or even older, and this premarital period is usually characterized by sexual adventures...." Men's later age at marriage seems to be an epiphenomenon of social expectations that men be able to support a family before they marry.

This expectation is true of Morocco, which, like parts of sub-Saharan Africa, is a polygamous society in which men and women inhabit separate spaces, but which is not usually described as sexually permissive or promiscuous. Fatima Mernissi (1983, 106), who studied sexual segregation, says of rural young men that most are indignant about feeling pushed into sexual practices—sodomy, homosexuality, and relations with prostitutes—which they abhor and which are proscribed by religion and custom. They dream of marrying, which they do as soon as they find a job; but in a country in which there is a high rate of unemployment, steady work is hard to find, and marriage is often delayed.

When Caldwell, Caldwell, and Quiggin (1989, 8ff.) refer to infidelity in the context of the AIDS epidemic, they are really concerned with women's sexual freedom, not with men's philandering. This is not the first time that women are the targets of an anti-venereal disease campaign. Yet it seems a bit late in the day to consider women's sexual behavior outside the context of women's economic conditions and social status, or to fail to consider the possibility that women's expression of their sexuality outside of wedlock is an act of resistance.

In societies in which marriage is nearly universal, in which poverty is extensive and living standards are low, in which educational opportunities are restricted, especially for girls, in which there are few job opportunities for young men, and even fewer for uneducated women, in which couples are frequently separated when men migrate in search of work, the sale of sexual services is likely to be common, blurring the line between infidelity and prostitution. There is an important feminist literature on prostitution in Europe and North America which places commercial sex work in its economic, social, and political context. These studies cast doubt on the claim that Africans are categorically different from "Eurasians" in this respect.

There is also a growing body of feminist work on prostitution in Africa to which Caldwell, Caldwell, and Quiggin make no reference. Luise White (1988, 139) makes the point that prostitution in Nairobi was domestic labor. In the colonial period, Kenyan men had access to waged work, women didn't; but men received only bachelor wages and were forced to migrate without their families. They paid prostitutes for domestic services, which included sleeping space, companionship, sexual relations, and food.

In these days of drastic structural adjustment policies when so much is being written about the failing economies of Africa, about falling standards of living, and the decline of health and education services, it is important to place the sale of sexual services in context. To search the anthropological literature for evidence of sexual permissiveness and promiscuity as inherent to African social organization adds insult to injury.

Caldwell, Caldwell, and Quiggin do not define the emotional bonds of marriage; they judge weakness by the frequency of divorce and extramarital relations. One should qualify this discussion with an exploration of intimacy in relation to sexuality. Three issues are relevant: the age difference between spouses, polygyny, and female circumcision. The first two are interrelated practices, which Caldwell, Caldwell, and Quiggin say reinforce weak conjugal bonds. Their third choice is postpartum sexual abstinence, a practice that appears to be disappearing; instead, it is useful to consider the custom of female circumcision.

Caldwell, Caldwell, and Quiggin (1989, 3-4) say that the great age gap between spouses reinforces the emotional and economic weakness of the conjugal bond. Certainly, an older man will exercise more authority and power over a young bride than a husband of her own age, but this is true whenever patriarchal relations exist and elders are respected; it is hardly unique to an alternative African civilization. In addition, the available data for Africa do not bear out the assertion that a great age gap exists everywhere.

Kaufmann, Lesthaeghe, and Meekers (1988, 225) in their study of six African countries found that for first marriages, men are three to eleven years older than women. The bigger age gap is typical of West Africa, especially the Islamic areas, but also of Kenya's Rift Valley and the Tswana, Ndebele, and Venda areas of South Africa. Elsewhere the gap is four to six years. An average age difference of four to six years is not striking, nor is it dissimilar to European custom. In France, the range is two to five years; the age gap takes the form of a U-shaped curve, with higher figures at both ends of the socioeconomic scale (INSEE 1987, 490).

Caldwell, Caldwell, and Quiggin consider polygyny to be the most distinctive feature of African marriage, made possible by the lack of stress on the need for a strong conjugal bond, which in turn does much to prevent such a strong bond from emerging, even in contemporary society. Polygyny, they continue, is "made possible by great pressure on widowed or divorced women to remarry quickly and by very substantial age gaps between spouses, typically ten years in the case of a man's first wife and decades with his youngest." (1989, 13) But polygyny is not unique to Africa—it is shared by Moslems the world over—nor is it universal in sub-Saharan Africa. Kaufmann, Lesthaeghe, and Meekers (1988, 225) say it is distributed in the same way as big age differences; it is common in West Africa, along the West African coast down to Angola, with less around the borders of Nigeria and Cameroon and between Côte d'Ivoire and Ghana, less among Sahelian nomads, even less in Central Africa, East Africa, and South Africa. It is higher (but still less than in West Africa) in a narrow zone extending from Kenya, Tanzania, Zambia, and Malawi, to Mozambique.

Does polygyny prevent strong conjugal bonds from emerging? Fainzang and Journet (1988) suggest that couples do form strong bonds in first marriages, which the arrival of a second wife can break. Mariama Bâ, in her poignant novel, *Une Si Longue Lettre*, writes eloquently of this situation. Women who object to a cowife may resist in two ways—either they flee, temporarily or permanently, when the rival arrives, or they withhold their savings to make it harder for their husband to accumulate the brideprice and thus forestall his second marriage (Fainzang and Journet 1988, 141).

First wives divorce less often than second or third wives, which suggests that these initial bonds are strong, even when they are founded on emotions other than romantic love.

It is interesting to compare North African and sub-Saharan data. Moroccan society shares some of the characteristics named by Caldwell, Caldwell, and Quiggin—polygynous households and an age gap between spouses. Namaane-Gessous (1988) is a Moroccan sociologist who studies sexuality. In the sample of women she interviewed, she found three distinct groups: the first was composed of women under thirty-five years of age with secondary or higher education for whom sex is pleasurable and an expression of love; a second group was composed of women over thirty-five with low levels of education for whom sex is a male affair—it leaves the women cold and calculating; a third group was composed of illiterate women over thirty-five who experience sex as an intolerable burden, a conjugal duty in return for which they are housed and fed. Couples in this last group share no affection, their marriage was arranged, and some of the women remember a brutal wedding night. The effects of education are evident in this sample, especially in the differences between generations, as more girls go to school and stay there longer. The data also suggest that the balance of power between men and women is changing, and that as women gain more equality, sexual intimacy deepens.

Namaane-Gessous has an interesting analysis of the lack of sexual intimacy in some marriages: poverty, especially in urban areas, deprives couples of privacy and of the time and space needed to create an intimate, erotic relationship. She quotes one woman as saying, "Since I married him we have lived in the same room as his mother. What can sexuality mean to me?" (1988, 212) Namaane-Gessous concludes that sensuality has little place in these older women's existence, and they don't necessarily miss it. To be desired by one's husband is a goal and a satisfaction in itself. And these women go to great lengths to remain the desired object.

In some parts of sub-Saharan African, circumcision is a prerequisite for marriage and only circumcised women are desirable.

They tell us that sex is dirty, taboo, you should be discreet if you talk about it. They also say that it is important to be faithful in marriage. Now, what is the justification of female circumcision? They think it diminishes sexual desire, so that means you will be faithful. They also say that female circumcision purifies women, that means that our sex genitalia is dirty....To them, female circumcision is very necessary to support their view of women's sexuality. (Assitan Diallo of Mali, quoted in Gevins 1987, 247)

Although they discuss postpartum sexual abstinence as a cause of weak emotional bonds, Caldwell, Caldwell, and Quiggin do not mention female circumcision, which is both a general health problem and a specific issue of sexuality (see Ladjali, Chapter Eight, for a discussion of the health issues). According to a 1979 estimate, 74 million, about one-third of all women in sub-Saharan Africa, have undergone some form of circumcision [2] (Paquot 1983, 339). An increasing number of African women are writing and speaking out about female circumcision (see, for example, Nawal El Saadawi, Asma El Dareer, Olayinka Koso-Thomas, and Awa Thiam). They seem to agree that this practice has lost its ritual significance of sexual initiation as it is now performed on infants and young children, and that it represents men's attempt to control women's sexuality, even though women perform the operation. This is a difficult subject to address, especially for non-Africans. Is female circumcision, which Ladjali suggests can be a psychologically and physically traumatic experience with lifelong consequences, a barrier to sexual equality and marital intimacy?

In some parts of sub-Saharan Africa, and not only in urban areas, young girls no longer passively accept parental disposition of their sexuality. Monimart (1989, 45) describes the changed behavior of uneducated teenagers with new options. The green bean fields of Lake Bam, Burkina Faso, provide a new source of revenue for young girls, fifteen to sixteen years old, who are able to earn enough to feed and clothe themselves. Contrary to tradition, they don't share their earnings with their parents, and they refuse to submit to parental authority. They claim sexual freedom to meet boys of their choice, without their parents' permission, and sometimes they become pregnant. Fearing a scandal, they try to hide their state as long as possible, but once it is known, they submit to their parents' will. Families that accept the illegitimate pregnancy try to find a husband for their daughter; those that do not accept it expel the girl, who will try to survive in the city.

In part these girls are rebelling against farm life in the Sahel, which desertification has made harder. It is more difficult to find water and firewood, it is necessary to walk longer distances in search of supplies, and the tendency is to carry heavier loads on the return journey so as to avoid making the long trips every day. Girls who work in the beanfields don't help their mothers with this arduous work.

This brings us to what Caldwell, Caldwell, and Quiggin term "the economic weakness of the conjugal bond" in sub-Saharan Africa. They cite two issues—that men and women maintain separate budgets, which they say reduces the economic unit to a woman and her children, and that there is a transactional element to sexual relations, even within marriage. One should review these issues in terms of household economies and control of labor, especially child labor.

Sex, Money, and Power in Marriage

Caldwell, Caldwell, and Quiggin (1989, 14-15) state that "transactions relating to sexual activity have been looked upon in Africa as equally normal as those relating to work" and that "the transactional element is widely present in marriage." There is a large body of Western literature on barter in marriage, including the plays of George Bernard Shaw, who commented upon this class-related phenomenon with broad sarcasm and delicious irony.

Dependent women necessarily bargain their unpaid labor, including sexual services, for household and personal expenses. Namaane-Gessous (1988) says that, in numerous couples, women take advantage of men's sexual desires to obtain items they need or want. She says that this attitude is particularly clear in polygynous households in which one wife obtains the goodwill or attachment of the husband by making herself more sexually available than another wife. This exchange is neither peculiar to Africa nor confined to polygynous societies in which the worlds of men and women are separate. From the male viewpoint, dependency is surely the strongest economic bond that can be forged.

Isn't the truth rather that men who hold economic power over women use it to obtain sexual favors from their wives and other women far more often than women use sex to obtain economic advantages from men? Namaane-Gessous (1988, 210) relates what a Moroccan woman told her: "If I refuse him, he will always find a way to take revenge; the next day, inventing some pretext, he will beat me, or very simply he will refuse to give me money for the marketing."

The central question here is whether African women are economically dependent or independent. Caldwell, Caldwell, and Quiggin (1989, 13) state that "in contemporary society [the African woman] is usually sufficiently economically independent that the dissolution of a marriage is not a financial disaster." This is a sweeping generalization for a continent composed of over fifty countries. In the diversity that is Africa, one can find examples of dependent and independent women. Fainzang and Journet (1988, 65) say that in both polygynous and monogamous Senegalese households, the husband customarily supplies daily, in money or kind, the food and new clothing needed that day. These men tie up their wives with a short rope! On the other hand, MacGaffey (1988) finds that some urban Zairian women are wealthy and that they successfully run lucrative businesses in the second economy, which escapes male control. Janet Jiggins (1989, 953) sums up the situation this way:

> In sub-Saharan Africa, household-based agricultural activity remains the foundation of rural livelihoods— and women do most of the work. Their activities are under increasing stress; they and their children are falling into poverty even as their need for cash income is increasing. Although they keep a foothold in the household economy, increasingly women are dependent on self-employment or wage work for survival; they have little access to services

and few opportunities to become more productive. Their situation is exacerbated by continuing male dominance and unequal household responsibilities. The informal sector offers opportunities for entrepreneurship, especially in trading or small-scale agroindustry, but unlicensed activity is discouraged in many countries. Some women also find themselves competing with businesses that are run or licensed by the state.

Roberts (1988) identifies access to labor as the key determinant of successful agricultural production in West Africa. Labor is a scarce resource, even in densely populated African countries (and most are still sparsely populated—in Nigeria, there are sixty-two inhabitants per square kilometer, in Côte d'Ivoire, there are seventeen, in Zaire, fourteen [*Etat du Monde* 1989]). Emerging from a number of West African studies reviewed by Roberts, and notably those by Jane Guyer, is the image of male heads of household who control the allocation of all labor at their command and of women who struggle for control of their own labor and that of their children. As Roberts (1988, 112) says, "When women cannot mobilize the labor of others they may work themselves to exhaustion."

Control over biological reproduction is not equal to control over the reproduction of the labor force and both are separate from the issue of who controls the allocation of labor. Human reproduction is not the same as reproduction of the labor force because not all children become workers: who works and who does which work are social decisions. The work of child rearing is also socially constituted; in Africa as elsewhere, it is consistently assigned to women. The child rearer, however, does not necessarily command the labor of the children she raises. In divorce, most women lose control of their children, who remain in the paternal household. Fathers may decide to send away some children, especially sons, for education. Nonetheless, many women find that their children provide the only assistance at their command, and one must ask whether this is an incentive to childbearing.

Stichter and Parpart (1988, 9) suggest that "children may be viewed as having both use value and exchange value under capitalist conditions." In Chapter Ten, Guillaume discusses the West African practice of foster care and details the extent to which children's labor power and their reproductive capacities have taken on exchange value in current capitalist conditions in Côte d'Ivoire. Women who foster girls not only profit from their labor but can expect to receive a child from their foster daughter after she marries; in effect, as grandmothers they will profit a second time from the child's labor.

One is easily tempted to collapse biological reproduction and reproduction of the labor force in Africa because children are put to work at a very early age. In the context of subsistence agriculture and domestic production, and in the absence of formal educational institutions, the aid that children give their parents may seem natural. The problems of child labor are not always recognized as such in Africa; some consider work to be part of children's socialization and not exploitation (Mendelievich 1980). But under capitalist conditions, children's use value can and does become exchange value.

Guillaume describes how fostering has changed in the current economic crisis. What began as a way for rural kin to offer their children an urban education became a way for the women who foster girls to obtain cheap domestic labor and a way for mothers to reduce the work of child rearing. In the current economic crisis, this practice has deteriorated further into the virtual sale of girls as domestics to unrelated families. Loewenson says in Chapter Three that men's employment on Zimbabwe plantations was sometimes made conditional upon the employment of their wives, and that children were also employed as cheap seasonal labor.

Monimart (1989, 42) describes the forced early marriage of girls in drought-stricken Mali for miserably low sums of bridewealth. Mothers told her of marrying their often very young daughters to the first man who offers to feed them and help the family. These marriages of misery are often ephemeral; after a few years, the young wife, abandoned or repudiated, returns to her parents, with one or two children in tow. One would think one was reading Pearl Buck's writings about pre-war, famine-stricken China, not present-day Africa. Fortunately, not all children are used in this way. Edholm, Harris, and Young (1977) are right to make the distinction between biological reproduction and reproduction of the labor force.

The Impact of Gender on Health

This chapter has attempted to portray health aspects of women's productive and reproductive labor in the broad framework of women's life experiences—marriage and divorce, sexuality and intimacy, submission and resistance—all of which take place in an economic, social, and political context of male-dominated institutions. The discussion is partial: it covers only the female gender and some, but not all, of women's health problems. The health services needed to address women's health problems are discussed in Chapter Twelve. Service needs should arise from problems, rather than from a logic internal to medical care or the political power of the medical profession; but not all health problems have medical or even public health solutions.

If millions of women risk their lives in unsafe abortions, curative services, such as free abortion on demand and surgical intervention (dilatation and curettage), are necessary, but as a response will be insufficient. Preventive measures, such as a choice of birth control methods and their concomitant counseling and medical supervision, are also needed, but they alone will not be sufficient. Women who derive recognition, a place in their households and communities, and some measure of security only from their status as wives and mothers, may not be able to use the contraceptives, or they may use them in secret and take enormous risks of reprisal.

The root of the problem is women's subordination and the limited opportunities African women have to gain recognition and independence through productive work. Education and training will help prepare them better for remunerative work, but shrinking economies offer few jobs. Explanations of the current economic crisis that blame economic failure on the lack of democracy (by which free-market economists mean open economies, not political freedoms) obfuscate the structural problems of the indenture to bankers and the abasement of the value of primary products, which African women are killing themselves to overproduce.

In summary, there are some women's health problems, such as female circumcision, which only African women can resolve, but there are a host of others arising from women's lack of control of their productive and reproductive labor, which demand solutions at the national and international level. Women of all nations, working in solidarity, can mount the pressures needed to bring about change.

· 8 ·

Conception, Contraception

Do Algerian Women Really Have a Choice?

MALIKA LADJALI*

BEFORE THE independence of Algeria in 1962, the concept of maternal and child health care did not exist. Health was not a recognized human right under French colonial rule. The care of mothers and children was a Christian act of charity, and the attitude that maternal and child health care is a charitable act continued after independence. The content of this charitable service was curative, because colonialists perceived the demand for curative care to be so great that they spent no time or money on preventive medicine. The first step in 1962 was to establish a national maternal and child health service, which included preventive care.

---

*Based on an interview and translation by Meredeth Turshen.

I began my career in maternal and child health in Algeria at a time when it was regarded as a positive field of work. Health was not a political term, and there was no social or governmental opposition to caring for the health of mothers and children; it was seen as a noble undertaking. Gradually, as I accumulated experience, other ideas followed. I wanted to integrate sexuality in maternal care. Later, the issue of women's rights arose in the context of human rights—women's rights to health information, education, services, and voluntary choice in childbearing. The United Nations eventually recognized these rights, but their translation into programs has been a veritable battle.

I use the terms family planning and contraception, rather than "reproductive health," because I find the latter too restrictive, too biological, too medical. "Reproductive health" evokes in us images of the uterus and the gynecologist. It is a negative term; one thinks not of health but of morbidity and mortality. And it excludes sexuality. We must invent a new term that reflects the woman's point of view. "Reproductive health" reflects the male physician's point of view.

In 1973 I took charge of maternal and child health services in Algeria and embarked on the second step to introduce family planning, which Algerians call *espacement des naissances*, birth or pregnancy spacing (Ladjali 1987). We began with only one family planning center, which the National Union of Algerian Women opened in 1967, and our problem was how to integrate family planning as an activity of maternal and child health services.

In keeping with my idea that family planning is a positive activity and not a medical one, I decided to retrain midwives to offer this service. Gynecologists were not ready to accept midwives in this role, despite the fact that they allowed midwives to assist in childbirth, which is after all a much more complicated procedure than the insertion of an intrauterine device. The designation of midwives as the key to the new family planning program was also a battle.

Even midwives were used to a curative, clinical practice in Algeria; it was a battle to persuade them that family planning is a broader concern of women, which must be situated in the context of their marriage and life in an extended family. Midwives needed to discover the woman in themselves and to think about birth control as an element of a woman's experience within a couple, in a rapidly changing society. This new perspective precipitated debates about women's roles among midwives and female physicians. The instructors were women physicians who also had to rethink the issues in order to teach the midwives. The medical profession is a masculine one, medical power is male, and medical training is a masculinizing experience for female medical students. Even women physicians have a man's attitude towards women patients. The retraining was so successful that women doctors who want an intrauterine device now consult midwives.

It took ten years to constitute teams of teachers for this course; eventually, the physicians were able to integrate sociologists, psychologists, and epidemiologists. Initially, the training took place in Algiers, but gradually it was decentralized. The training course lasted one month and included both practical and theoretical components.

We have now made available several types of contraception; even women in rural areas have a choice. Access to maternal and child health and family planning services had been geographically limited in rural areas, but it has gradually been improved. This is not to say that women in urban areas have no problems. The woman who is stuck in low-income housing and cannot leave home until evening when her husband returns from work, by which time the clinic is closed, does not have easy access to family planning. Young women do not go out alone, and the only transport available may be an expensive taxi, which they cannot afford.

And once the woman—urban or rural—is in the health system, what choice does she really have? Do technical options really represent choice? Or are there cultural constraints on women's ability to use contraception?

Why Women Accept or Reject Contraception

We spoke initially in the Algerian program of the *offer* of family planning; only later did we come to ask ourselves about the *demand* for family planning. Together with Claudine Chaulet, professor of sociology at the University of Algiers, we studied the demand for contraception (Ladjali and Chaulet 1985). We were aware that Algerian women were changing and that village traditions no longer monopolized the regulation of childbearing. For example, some of the salient changes that have occurred in the past generation are civil registration of birth, childbirth in a hospital, the vaccination of children, the growing preference of young people to form nuclear families, the choice by some women not to marry, and the emergence of women who head households. Clearly, the principle that couples can choose the number of children they have and the intervals at which they have them has found its place in the process of family adaptation to current realities.

We wondered, then, not only about the women who came for family planning services, but also about the women who did not come. If we wanted to attract women to our services, we had to use arguments that were based on compassion and a solid comprehension of the cultural and institutional foundations of their lives.

On reflection we realized that the rejection of contraception has several motives. One pattern is the outright rejection of the idea by the husband, his wife, and the extended family, who understand family planning as a sin. No economic rationale for birth control has an impact on this position, which is reinforced by social realities. The extended family functions as a cohesive unit, combining income and resources. It follows that the strongest and most influential families are those with the most sons. So long as adult sons find work, large numbers of children will be experienced as a strength and not as a weakness. Indeed, an economic rationale can backfire: the poorest families will resent the injustice of the wealthy being able to have as many children as they want, whereas the poor must deprive themselves of the only hope and happiness they are allowed. Absolute refusal of contraception can also be understood as a claim for autonomy from state interference in intimate family affairs.

Sometimes the refusal came from the husband, whereas the wife wanted to control her fertility. In some of these cases, the husband feared that birth control would compromise his social image, and he may have been supported by his mother who controls his wife's daily life. The birth of a child demonstrates that a man is not impotent, which may be very important to someone whose social position is low or who has been unable to realize his ambitions. In other cases, the husband sought through successive births to prove his authority over the entire family, whose honor must be unimpeachable; such a husband may have seen the practice of contraception by his wife (and the regulation of fertility is almost always a woman's affair in Algeria) as her way of evading his control.

When a woman said to a midwife who offered contraception that her husband has not given his permission, she may have been expressing the belief that she must fulfill an unwritten contract to bear many children. Some mothers insisted on the legitimacy of their position by complaining about their fatigue and misery. These women were responsive to health rationales for family planning, when the service was readily available and offered discreetly in the context of care for their health and the health of their children.

Some women themselves refused family planning, and their rejection had to be understood in the context of the Algerian cultural system, which dictates that children are a woman's only legitimate happiness, her only way to attain a respected status in her husband's family. (Traditionally, an Algerian woman lives with her husband's family, under the thumb of her mother-in-law; in time, her sons will bring their brides [whom she will choose] to live with her, and her adult sons will ensure her survival in old age.) By bearing and raising many children, a woman demonstrates her courage and acquires dignity.

The women in this group expressed no desire to space pregnancies at the beginning of their marriage. They considered the first births to be a blessing, and they experienced their infants as a joy. Pregnancies were naturally spaced by prolonged breastfeeding, during which the mothers enjoyed physical contact with their babies and followed their development with tenderness. Any feeling that young children were a burden was usually lessened in the extended family by the presence of several women with children of various ages. Women in this situation who rejected contraception sometimes complained about the inability to provide all of the things their children needed, but they did not protest the number of children they had.

Only later, when these women had already raised many children including several sons, did they bring up the question of contraception. Only after they had fulfilled their marriage contract, proven their courage in childbirth, and assured their status, could these women pay attention to their worries about family finances and their own fatigue. Even then, birth control was not envisaged as an irreversible process because there was too much physical insecurity and uncertainty about the future.

Infant mortality is still too high in Algeria—81 per 1,000 live births in 1985—to permit women to believe that all of their babies will survive. Nor does the law, and even less social custom, guarantee a woman's social status, which traditionally depends upon her sons; this insecurity is aggravated by the new trend to form nuclear families, which is at odds with traditional values of family cohesion and collective survival strategies. Also, to end childbearing is to age socially, to pass into another role, which not all women (who may be only thirty-five years old by the time they have had five or six children) are prepared to do. With posterity assured, however, a consensus may emerge and the couple may agree to use birth control. (The technical response is imperfect, since few methods guarantee a reversible interruption of childbearing.) This situation of older couples with many children describes most of the demand for family planning in Algeria today.

Listening to Algerian Women

Several points emerge from this consideration of women's reasons to reject contraception. It is evident that structural conditions for the general and rapid acceptance of contraception do not yet exist in Algeria, but the diffusion of information that takes into account women's social realities can spread the practice. For example, ethnic and religious traditions rigidly separate the lives of women and men and dictate modest behavior for women in the presence of their fathers, brothers, and husbands. But within masculine and feminine circles, sexual matters are openly discussed with no prudery. So long as the separation of the sexes is respected, schools and health institutions can offer sex education classes that give explicit instruction on contraception.

This is what we mean when we say that we must listen to women's needs and expectations for family planning services that are readily available and offered discreetly in the context of maternal and child health care. In a society in which men and women live apart, women develop intense solidarity among themselves, despite occasional rivalries. Among women of the same generation, complicity is immediate in everything concerning motherhood; a living culture of exchanges and mutual support grows up around the children. If inserted within women's relationships, the idea of consulting a midwife for help in spacing pregnancies can be successfully diffused.

Contraception that is in the hands of women (users and providers) and not excessively medicalized can be integrated into women's search for new models of behavior. Algerian women are in the process of redefining themselves in their daily lives and social roles. The most spectacular changes—education and waged work—are part of a transformation that touches women of all social classes. For example, the purchase of manufactured goods that were formerly produced at home has transformed domestic work; and the role of consumer gives women a new basis for their status in the family. Now that they have a budget to manage, women must learn how to make rational purchases. Schools and health clinics have transformed women's traditional roles as educators and nurses of their children; at the same time, these institutions have created new tasks. Women are learning how to support their children at school so that they will be sucessful. Educated mothers are becoming active agents of their children's advancement at school, and they value the instruction given to their daughters because it may help their future grandchildren.

This transformation of women's lives, the opportunity it offers women to assume different functions, also provides a new basis for a couple's consensus. The future of their children, knowing what strategies to pursue to ensure a child's advancement, mobilizes parental energies and becomes a meeting point for mothers and fathers. If it can be proven that it is less difficult to help children when there are fewer of them, the couple may reach an agreement to adopt contraception, not as an egotistical measure to ease the parents' lives, but as a benevolent measure taken for the good of their children.

As providers of health and contraceptive services, we needed to take the transformation of women's lives into account on a very practical basis. For example, before independence it was the French colonial custom to open public services in the morning and to offer private care in the afternoon. We maintained that practice, without considering that it is precisely in the morning that women's workload is heaviest and that women have the least free time to attend a clinic.

We needed to think about the effect of health activities on family planning, and not only the effect of family planning on health activities. Women who had a positive attitude toward maternal and child health clinics because they brought their children to them to be vaccinated were among the first to come for family planning when the service was presented as a health measure.

We needed to offer better care in pregnancy and childbirth—more frequent prenatal consultations and more attention to premature births—in order to help more newborns survive. One-third of infant mortality occurs in the first month after birth, but most maternal and child health care activities focus on the problems of infants from the second through the eleventh month, when two-thirds of deaths occur. The ability to intervene surgically during difficult births would save many lives.

Our responses to Algerian women's health problems were fivefold. First was the program to retrain midwives to listen to women—for example, to look after the comfort of the woman in childbirth (and not only the welfare of the newborn)—and to respond to women as women.

Second was a study of the quality of care, as distinguished from the quantity of services, which was already the subject of much family planning research. There are few indicators to measure or evaluate the quality of care. Family planning is usually regarded as a technical service requiring quantitative analysis. Yet we are aware, for example, that the women most in need of counseling are the least likely to receive it and vice versa, that the women who are already educated and working outside the home are most likely to receive extensive counseling. I distinguish here between information conveyed by mass media, education conducted in small groups, and one-on-one counseling. Economic class plays an important role in the demand and offer of counseling.

Our third response was to undertake operational research, which would give us quick results. Operational research must be carried out in third world countries such as Algeria. Falsely, the urgency of dispensing health care and the high cost of research are always cited as reasons for not doing any research in the third world. If third world professionals are not integrated into research projects, it is hardly surprising that third world women are not integrated into primary health care.

This brings us to our fourth point: that women must participate in primary health care. The current situation is aggravated by the attitude of professionals trained in biomedicine who equate traditional practices with harmful practices and who make women clients feel guilty about their customs. It is not true that all traditional practices are harmful. We need to validate those customs that are beneficial. And we need to associate women in the definition of primary health care.

Finally, literacy is usually offered as an activity that is separate from women's daily concerns. Instead of listening to what it is that women would like to learn—how to write their names? how to read their child's weight chart? how to add and subtract?— educational programs make women feel ignorant. Health professionals laugh when a woman comes into a clinic and spreads out all the family documents because she cannot distinguish her child's health card from her marriage certificate. Our proposal is to tie literacy projects to the content of primary health care.

When an illiterate, uneducated woman is given a prescription for the Pill without any counseling about side effects or alternatives, her body is in effect offered to the medical service. Rather than giving her control of her reproductive functions, the family planning service is in reality violating her. A prescription for the Pill is written more quickly than an intrauterine device can be inserted; if service personnel are pressed for time and give women the Pill, can we say this is women's choice? If the use of intrauterine devices is low in Algeria, Morocco, and Tunisia, is it because North African women prefer the Pill, or because they are offered the Pill as sole option? If service personnel took more time to counsel each woman, would the Pill be her first choice? Educated women who have had an opportunity to talk with health professionals, who have read more and have questions to ask, use intrauterine devices more often; they can impose their choice on service personnel, unlike illiterate women who must accept whatever the staff propose.

Our reflections about the demand for family planning led us to ask about the determinants of conception and contraception. First, we needed to specify which women we were talking about: middle-aged women with five children? the young waged worker? the woman who has remained in her natal village? or the one who was raised in Algiers? Does it make sense to respond to the millions of women who come to family planning clinics with the same menu of Pills, intrauterine devices, and sterilization? Each woman bears a cultural heritage and harbors anguished, contradictory questions about contraception.

Secondly, we looked at how motivation was the greatest single determinant of birth control. At some level, motivation was the same in every case. When a couple did not want a child, even without contraception, there was no pregnancy. When a child was wanted, even with the Pill, the woman became pregnant. Motivation is an individual characteristic, but in certain circumstances it can be thwarted. For example, there was a woman who had had three daughters in three difficult pregnancies and did not want any more children, but her motivation was overtaken by her mother-in-law who insisted on a grandson.

Demographic Concerns

In 1986, the Algerian family planning program took on a new function: to lower the national birth rate. The change entailed was dramatic. Family planning involves only the medical corps, which promotes health as a rationale for contraception. But contraception is only one aspect of fertility. A population control program involves many other aspects of fertility; for example, it has economic and cultural aspects, which ministries other than the health ministry must take into account. Family planning entails individual counseling; population control employs mass media campaigns, in which the health rationale is no longer primary. The difference between family planning and population control lies in the huge difference between contraceptive use and fertility control.

When a population control campaign praises the two-child family, for example, it appeals to a sense of sacrifice and makes women with more than two children—and women who want more than two children—feel guilty. This message does not motivate women to have smaller families, nor does it help them deal with their anxieties. Or to give another example, many women refuse contraception because of the side effects. These side effects reflect a woman's state of mind and cannot be dismissed as imaginary. Only a male doctor would describe depression, daily headaches, and weight gain as minor side effects. Women's reproductive organs elicit emotionally charged reactions; if women are not able to express these feelings, they may convert their psychological reactions into physical complaints. Or look at the Pill, which really signifies a part of the woman herself. Its daily ingestion is not like swallowing an aspirin—its implications are much greater—yet it is represented as medication and prescribed by a doctor.

Mass media antinatalist campaigns publicize sexuality along with contraception; this can be a brutal confrontation for the modest woman who has been brought up to repress her sexual feelings and to regard her body as belonging, not to herself, but to her father, brothers, and husband. Publicity campaigns, in this cultural context, violate women's privacy and make them feel uneasy. To change attitudes about having children is not as simple as distributing contraceptives; if it were, contraception would have been practiced as widely and for as long as breastfeeding has been.

The public campaign for population control was successful in Algeria and had some positive effects. It did result in a larger demand for contraceptives. We may ask, was it due to the campaign's message or to the freedom women felt to express a desire they had been harboring for a long time? The antinatalist campaign changed the public image of the woman who practices family planning, and this may have permitted some women to come forward who had been afraid of the public reaction to their having no more children.

The approach to family planning in Algeria is different from that in Morocco and Tunisia. These three North African countries share many cultural values such as the Islamic faith and the pattern of extended families. The Algerian family planning program is governmental, the Tunisian program is parastatal, and in Morocco, nongovernmental organizations and the private sector play important roles in the program. Tunisia was the first of the three countries to inaugurate family planning, the only Arab country to legalize abortion; it has outlawed polygamy and banned repudiation as a man's means of divorcing his wife. Despite these differences, the results of the family planning programs are remarkably similar: in all three countries, 30 to 40 percent of women use some form of contraception.

The Tunisian program is the oldest, dating from 1964; it is an aggressive antinatalist campaign. Recent studies show that such campaigns do not play a decisive role in reducing the birthrate. There are other determinants such as later age at marriage and the suppression of polygamy, which have a greater impact. We have placed too much emphasis on contraception without examining what determines a couple's childbearing behavior and how to change it. The problem of providing family planning in North Africa cannot be compared with the questions that confront the developed countries. In advanced industrial countries, maternity is one of women's many life choices, and the question is how to place contraception within everyone's reach. In North Africa, motherhood is often the only role women can play in society.

A population control program that relies upon contraception alone will have limited success in our countries. These campaigns try to influence the demand for contraception when what they need to influence is the continuous and long-term use of contraception. A global study shows that 50 percent of the world's women know about contraception but only half of them use it. Modern contraception is an imported technology that will be absorbed slowly.

Later age at marriage is a striking trend in all three North African countries. According to a national study carried out in Algeria, the average age at marriage in 1986 was 23.8 years for women and 27.6 years for men (ENAF 1987). There is surprisingly little difference in rural areas, in which the figures are 22.7 years for women and 26.4 years for men. Studies in Tunisia show that later age at marriage has had more impact on the birthrate than has the family planning program. Other social influences are the increasing number of girls enrolled in primary school and the extension of health services. Both general mortality and infant mortality rates are falling in the three countries.

Abortion is not legal in Algeria, nor is adoption. If an unmarried woman becomes pregnant, she—not the father—will be blamed. Her only recourse is to give birth in another town and to abandon the child in an orphanage. In addition to the psychological trauma of birth and separation from her child, the young mother is burdened by the knowledge that orphanages do not provide a nurturing environment. Tunisia, unlike Algeria and Morocco, authorizes both abortion and adoption, with the result that there are few abandoned children in Tunisia today (Ennaïfer 1988).

Algeria shares cultural values with its neighbors to the east and west, but historically it is also affiliated with countries to the south. In my travels through sub-Saharan Africa, I am struck by strong differences in attitudes toward sexuality, virginity, illegitimacy, and circumcision.

There is an openness about sexuality, even in the Muslim parts of sub-Saharan Africa, that is absent in North Africa, where women's place is differently defined. There appears to be no public taboo on sexuality in the parts of sub-Saharan Africa that I visited. Virginity does not seem to have the same cultural value; in North Africa, virginity defines and circumscribes a girl's life from the time she is born to the day she marries (Naamane-Gessous 1988). In Zaire, for example, no one seems to worry if a woman has one or two children before she marries. (In countries in which sexually transmitted diseases are the cause of widespread sterility, proof of fertility before marriage is desirable.) As a result of these differences, there are no abandoned children; no social problems surround illegitimacy in Francophone countries south of the Sahara. Family planning is rarely practiced, but then few family planning services are available. In some countries, 1 percent of couples use contraception; in Nigeria the figure is 6 percent and in Kenya it is 18 percent. These figures are low; in comparison, over 30 percent of North African couples practice family planning.

Female Circumcision

The practice of female circumcision affects millions of women, most of them in sub-Saharan Africa. Performed as a cultural rite, circumcision is not required by any religion. Female circumcision is not practiced in Algeria, Morocco, or Tunisia. It is one of many traditional practices that affect women's health, some positively, some negatively; it should not be considered in isolation from other traditional practices. Cicumcision must be seen in the context of the very heavy burden of disease and poor health conditions that exist in Africa—for example, widespread malnutrition and malaria, early pregnancy and the unavailability of Caesarean sections during difficult births. Cicumcision also should be seen as a changing problem within a dynamic society. For the past ten years, African women have been working on this question. They train, they educate, they inform, and they voice their feelings. African leaders in Benin, Burkina Faso, Kenya, and Senegal, among others, have made public statements condemning the practice, and in 1978, Egypt passed a law banning it. In 1984, an Inter-African Committee (IAC) was created to study the problem: it now has national committees in sixteen countries and is coordinating research in nine of them (Ladjali and Toubia 1990).

Can the efforts of African and Arab women be reinforced by creating a space for counseling, a free space for those who suffer or have silent unanswered questions about female circumcision? To answer this question, I traveled to Nigeria and Mali.

There are three types of female circumcision: the first, known in Muslim countries as Sunna circumcision, involves the removal of the foreskin of the clitoris, simulating male circumcision; the second, excision, involves the removal of a part or all of the clitoris, together with a part or all of the labia minora; and the third, infibulation (also known as pharaonic circumcision), the most severe form, involves in addition to excision, removal of the medial parts of the labia majora, joining the two sides of the vulva, and leaving only a small hole through which urine and menstrual fluids pass.

Surgery in the genital area carries risks, especially when it is performed without anesthesia and with a razor blade, knife, or a straw. Female circumcision has immediate and long-term complications that can result in physical and psychological damage. Immediate risks include bleeding, tetanus, infection, septicemia, and death. HIV infection can be contracted from the instruments used for cutting. Extreme pain and shock owing to the lack of anesthesia may also occur. The long-term side effects pose general and specific health problems: severe scarring and chronic infections of the kidneys and urinary tract, sterility, coital difficulty, infection, pregnancy loss, and complications during childbirth. Psychological damage is associated with the strong feelings of threat, anguish, and anxiety that surround surgery on the genital organs. Female circumcision has a powerful impact on the psychosexual development and self-image of the little girl and later woman. Mental disturbances resulting from circumcision are unlikely to find a remedy in an environment that has created them.

Attempts to eradicate this practice have taken many routes, with varying degrees of success. Among the many lessons learned, the most important are that people cannot be forced into social change by passing laws, that those who are aware of the harm must work with the community for change, and that women are not victims of just circumcision: they face a plethora of health, economic, and social problems. Attempts to combat circumcision should be incorporated into wider efforts to improve women's status.

The tradition of dialogue with women about contraception can be adapted to help women who suffer from the real and deep pains of mutilation. Care for these women should be integrated in counseling, and their suffering should be acknowledged by appropriately trained staff. For this purpose, family planning associations should create spaces with an atmosphere in which women feel free, are listened to, and can express their innermost fears and concerns about female circumcision.

In addition to contact with sub-Saharan Africa, Algeria retains strong ties to France. The Mediterranean separates North Africa from Europe, but it also describes a unifying culture dating back to ancient Egypt, Greece, and Rome. Whatever the history, today Europe is two hours away by air, and there are six daily flights between Algiers and Paris (all of them full). In addition to the French colonial impact, which includes a tradition of labor migration, European influence is felt through radio and television programs and, in Tunisia and Morocco, through the tourist trade. This proximity poses many questions of national identity and problems of adaptation. It is troubling that North African women are faced with a whole range of new decisions—everything from consumerism in supermarkets to choices for their children—without any public debate or discussion about women's changing role in society.

An Algerian woman who lives in France confronts a pronatalist discourse—the French encourage childbearing by paying a benefit for each child (*allocation familiale*), for example. Pronatalist practices are in direct conflict with the antinatalist campaign in Algeria. On the other hand, the migrant may be encouraged to try Depo-Provera, an injectable hormonal contraceptive administered every three months that is not available in Algeria. On her visit home, she may boast about it as a mark of her new status, along with her new clothes, gifts, and French vocabulary. If this boast creates a demand for Depo-Provera among village women, the Algerian health service will not be able to respond. It cannot train staff fast enough to provide conventional contraception, and Depo-Provera requires more medical follow-up than other methods.

A separate issue is the cultural dislocation of child rearing practices: an Algerian mother in France will encounter an indifferent attitude toward the virginity of her daughter at the maternal and child health clinic. She may try to enlist the aid of an uncomprehending doctor in obtaining a certificate of virginity demanded by the family of her daughter's fiancé.

These are just some of the problems; I have discussed only a few of the social questions surrounding family planning, which face the woman who migrates to Europe. Interested readers are referred to Lacoste-Dujardin (1986), who discusses more of them at length.

A Woman's Space

Women's sexuality is a complex issue; to unravel it, women need time and space. I would so much like to see the maternal and child health clinic become a woman's space where women talk about their health, the problems and joys of raising children, and their lives as women. Open all day, the clinic would offer all the services that women need. The clinic managers and staff would be women-conscious and listen to women seriously. I would like the clinic to be a place that does not make women feel guilty about mistakes they make in raising their children, a place that values all positive traditional practices. Historically, women were the healers and educators of their families; we should not turn this advantage into a guilt trip because a woman fails to sterilize a bottle correctly or misses a vaccination date. I would like to see clinic staff teach women to recognize when they need to seek medical care for themselves, their children, and their families.

To listen to women, to value them in their roles as wives and mothers, to offer services by women, for women, and also with them—that is my dream for maternal and child health and family planning services.

· 9 ·

The Politics of Population Control in Namibia

JENNY LINDSAY

IN THE EARLY 1970s, when Namibia was still under South African control, the South African government implemented a national family planning program in South Africa (Brown 1987; Edmunds 1981; Gray 1980) and subsequently extended it to Namibia. The government funded the Namibian program extensively and provided free contraception throughout the country; family planning was the only free health service it provided. There was no public discussion of the program, although a letter printed in the *South African Journal of Medicine* in 1976 gave an account of the way in which it was set up in the capital city of Windhoek and its success in bringing down the birthrate of indigent people (Orford 1976). Whether it is necessary to reduce the birthrate in a territory that is roughly the size of France and the British Isles put together, that has a population of two million (at most), and that has a birthrate of 2.5, has not been adequately demonstrated, either then or since.

South Africa and Namibia implemented a state policy of population control, as opposed to family planning. The term "population control" covers family planning programs as well as broad policies designed to control population movement and to restrict migration (Brown 1987); for example, it includes South Africa's policy to keep the black and white populations separate by restricting Africans to certain designated areas. Policies designed to control women's fertility are the most recent manifestation of long-standing population control policies. These newer policies are particularly sinister because they masquerade as well-meaning family planning programs intended to alleviate poverty by reducing the numbers of children. Policies intended to reduce unwanted pregnancies are qualitatively different from earlier policies, which were strategies for acquiring cheap labor and controlling its movement.

South African policies were designed to reduce the black populations of South Africa and Namibia. In 1987 Moses Katjiuongua, minister of health and welfare in the puppet administration, perpetuated the idea that "unbridled population growth is the most serious problem facing South West Africa [sic] today." He also referred to a statement by a right-wing political leader, Sarl Becker, who, in a public meeting in Mariental, urged the white population to outdo the black population in "baby production."

There is no doubt that many women do wish to exercise control over the size of their families and that they welcome access to contraception, but they also wish to choose when to use contraception and the kind of contraception to use. They need information to enable them to make meaningful choices, however, and they need guidance from a medical profession they can trust. The issues discussed here are complicated and, in Namibia, involve a struggle for control over fertility, not simply between men and women, nor simply between classes, but between a dominant white elite and a section of a subordinate black working class that is made up of black women.

Women's personal experience, both as patients and nurses, is the primary focus of this research, and much of the data consists of interviews with women, both in groups and individually. Before independence in March 1990, there was a lack of official documentation of any meaningful kind in Namibia, and a reluctance on the part of the South African administration to divulge information. As a result, this study relies heavily on oral sources. Most of the interviews were prearranged group encounters with women in urban areas, even in the north of Namibia. During the first visit in 1983, I began by interviewing women in the black township of Katatura, just outside the capital city of Windhoek. Detailed interviews with key informants in the community such as nurses, teachers, and social workers, enabled me to place myself in the situation as they perceived it. These early interviews were open-ended, allowing women to express their interests and concerns. Subsequent interviews were arranged with women of all ages, not educated in European-style schools, and not necessarily English-speaking. These group discussions were lively, as women exchanged information with each other, appealed to each other for advice or further information, and considered strategies for dealing with the problems of everyday life. I interviewed women from Ovamboland and Kavango, women of Herero, Nama, and Damara ethnic groups, and women of mixed origins (classified as "coloreds" by South Africa). During the second and third visits in 1985 and 1986, I concentrated on interviewing nurses and physicians in departments of gynecology and obstetrics and nurses in family planning clinics.

Contraception is provided largely in the form of Depo-Provera injections in Namibia. The long-term effects of these hormonal injections are still unknown, but Depo-Provera is banned by the Food and Drug Administration in the United States because there is evidence that connects the drug with various forms of cancer, in particular cervical cancer (WHO 1984). In Namibia, the black population is the program's target; hospital personnel administer injections immediately after childbirth, often without the woman's consent or knowledge, and family planning personnel give women injections in family planning clinics throughout the country. In Katatura, the black township of Windhoek, the common dosage is 450 milliliters, three times the usual, normal, or standard dosage

(Orford 1976). The effects of such massive doses are simply unknown.

The questions raised here are of importance to the women of Namibia. How they are answered is a matter for the Namibian people to decide in the light of their own discussions. The information brings to light a hidden form of oppression that may have long-term effects. Central to this research project is the belief that the women who have had Depo-Provera tested upon them have the right to be heard, and this study allows them to speak out and give their own evidence.

Namibian Women's Experience of Depo-Provera

Throughout Namibia women report widespread coercion in state facilities. In the words of one black Namibian physician, Depo-Provera injections are "simply banged into black and colored women, without discussion, explanation or even permission." (Interview, Windhoek, October 1983). In Katatura, women interviewed confirmed that Depo-Provera injections are given on the labor wards after delivery and that patients are afforded little opportunity for informed consent or refusal. Even allowing for misunderstandings due to language problems and the difficulties in communication when patients and hospital staff do not speak the same language, the stories are common enough to be taken very seriously. Three stories illustrate the difficulties women faced in Katatura Hospital.

A woman tells of her experience after the birth of her first child:

> After my son was born in the hospital here the nurse gave me an injection. I wasn't ill so I wondered what it was for and I asked the nurse later on. She told me it was Depo-Provera, to prevent me having another baby. I was really angry because I wanted another child. I didn't want an injection. (Interview, Katatura, October 1983)

A mother tells of her experience with two daughters:

My first daughter went into hospital to have her baby, and they gave her a Depo-Provera injection without asking for her consent and without her knowledge, after she delivered. Afterwards she suffered continuous bleeding, which had to be treated with pills and it was a terrible experience for her. Later my younger daughter also gave birth in Katatura Hospital and they put pressure on her to have a Depo-Provera injection. They told her that she could not leave hospital until she had had an injection. I went there and told them that she was leaving and that we already had enough trouble with those injections. So she left hospital without an injection. (Interview, Katatura, October 1983)

A young woman explains that the nurse gave her an injection after the birth of her first child: "I only had one child but she did not seem to think that mattered. I thought they only gave you injections if you already had a big family." (Interview, Windhoek, October 1983)

Routine injections after childbirth, when women are most vulnerable, is one of the most insensitive features of the family planning campaign. Evidence obtained from women in the black township directly contradicts assurances by the physician in charge, Dr. Orford, that postpartum injections are not given. Accounts of exactly what happens in Katatura Hospital vary but evidence from all of the twenty-three nurses interviewed confirms that patients are routinely given Depo-Provera injections directly after childbirth. The data sheet published in England by Upjohn, the sole manufacturer of Depo-Provera, expressly advises against this practice: "If the puerperal woman will be breastfeeding, the initial injection should be delayed until six (6) weeks postpartum, when the infant's enzyme is more developed."

Pressure to comply and accept the injections is strong, as one nurse explained: "Women are not accustomed to asking questions or contradicting whites, and peasant women are not likely to contradict professional women such as nurses." (Interview,

Windhoek, February 1985) Stories of women given Depo-Provera injections without their knowledge are commonplace in Katatura. One nurse told this story about an Ovambo woman who came to see her:

> When she left hospital after the birth of her last child she was issued with a card and asked to return in three months' time. She was quite confused by this and came to ask me about it and why she was asked to return. When I told her she had been given a contraceptive injection she was shocked because she certainly would not have had such an injection as she wanted another child. (Interview, Windhoek, February 1985)

There is no means of knowing how extensive the routine administration of postpartum contraceptive injections is, but the interview evidence suggests indiscriminate administration of Depo-Provera to women in the hospital, regardless of their medical history, the present size of their family, or personal circumstances. For example, during a discussion with a group of women one nurse remarked:

> I know a woman who had one child and went into hospital to have a second child after fourteen years. They gave her a Depo-Provera injection immediately after she had delivered. You couldn't say she had too many children, could you? But that's what they keep on telling us, that we have too many children. (Interview, Katatura, October 1983)

Two other young women in the same group complained that they had been given injections immediately after the birth of their first child, without being asked for their permission: neither wanted the injection.

Occasionally, women who have not had a child are given Depo-Provera injections arbitrarily, without any kind of consultation. A physician related this story:

A married woman in her early twenties went into Katatura Hospital with a miscarriage and was afterwards given the standard three-month Depo-Provera injection without her permission, and thus rendered infertile for more than a year. They didn't care about the psychological need for her to conceive again as soon as possible. (Interview, Windhoek, February 1985)

This same physician stated that hospital and clinic staff in Katatura and Khomasdal family planning clinics even ignore physicians' letters with specific recommendations. Patients for whom one physician recommended the fitting of a Copper T intrauterine device or the provision of Pills returned saying, "She just gave me the injection anyway." (Interview, Windhoek, February 1985)

Hospital patients are particularly liable to receive contraceptive injections as part of their treatment, and interviews with patients and with nurses in Katatura seem to indicate that Depo-Provera injections are a regular feature of state care. Women suffering from tuberculosis have been coerced into receiving Depo-Provera injections. One nurse reported that the physician with whom she worked often refused patients treatment unless they agreed to have contraceptive injections, often "chasing women away" when they were seriously ill. (Interview, London, 1985). In early 1985 all female patients in the tuberculosis wards in Katatura Hospital were receiving contraceptive injections, except one nine-year old girl, but including a woman who had already had a hysterectomy (Interview, Windhoek, February 1985). The physicians' rationale is that the drugs administered in the treatment of tuberculosis are dangerous for pregnant women, but this information is not communicated to the women. Instead, the following scenario is typical: a young married teacher who had never had a child found that she was suffering from tuberculosis. She fully understood the problems a pregnancy would pose and wished to continue to take contraceptive Pills as she had always done. The doctor failed to inform her that anti-TB drugs block the metabolism of the Pill, rendering it ineffective and exposing her to pregancy; he simply forced her to have Depo-Provera injections as part of her treatment.[1] (Interview, Katatura, February 1985)

Mental patients are also given Depo-Provera injections while they are in the hospital and these injections are usually continued after they have been discharged. One woman interviewed, distressed by massive and unhealthy weight gain due to the injections, said that she did not dare to complain. A mobile van came to take her to the hospital regularly every three months and she feared that they would hospitalize her again if she refused to have the injections. (Interview, Windhoek, February 1985).

Abortion is illegal in Namibia as in South Africa, but in January 1985 the abortion wards in Katatura Hospital were full (thirty-six patients in all). All of these women were given contraceptive injections before being allowed to leave and were in no position to refuse.

Depo-Provera: The Side Effects

Most Namibian women with experience of Depo-Provera, voluntary or otherwise, complain of side effects that are often sufficiently unpleasant to discourage them from continuing the injections. Nurses and patients mention two major side effects: complete cessation of menstrual bleeding (amenorrhea), which the women find disconcerting and unnatural; or, worse still, nonstop bleeding, which, not surprisingly, they find quite intolerable. One woman said: "I had just one injection, and afterwards I was bleeding all the time. It went on for more than a year. It was really terrible. I won't have another injection. I think the coil sounds better and I might try that." (Interview, Katatura, November 1983)

Decrease in sexual interest was also mentioned frequently. Perhaps those who consider this a small price to pay for freedom from pregnancy might consider whether this is a price that most men would be prepared to pay. Certainly many women in Katatura were not happy about this particular accompaniment to contraceptive injections and there was some evidence that their disinterest in sex caused marital problems. A social worker reported:

This man I have just seen has marital problems. He told me that his wife lost interest in sex since she started having

Depo-Provera injections. I suggested that he should use some form of contraception instead of his wife but he was outraged at that suggestion. He told me that he's looking for another woman. (Interview, Katatura, February 1985)

Another woman spoke sadly of the decrease in sexual desire after Depo-Provera injections: "I don't have a boyfriend any more. I have no feeling for a man these days." (Interview, Katatura, November 1983) However this woman, who already had six children, said that the decrease in sexual feeling was the price she was prepared to pay for freedom from pregnancy: "I was so relieved when I discovered Depo-Provera injections. I can't afford to be pregnant any more. I have to keep my children, and I can't afford to have any more."

Long-term effects of Depo-Provera are now beginning to appear. According to physicians and nurses interviewed in the north of Namibia in 1983 and 1985, many women who were given Depo-Provera injections during the 1970s when they were young and who subsequently decided to start a family or to have more children, are having difficulties in conceiving. Physicians are worried about the number of such women coming for gynecological help, and worried too about the continuing use of Depo-Provera and the implications for the future. Women interviewed reported waiting four, five, and six years to have a child. Treatment for infertility is costly and out of reach of many women: "My sister and I had Depo-Provera injections in the early seventies. It cost me four hundred rand before I succeeded in giving birth to my son after three years. My sister, whom you have just seen with her little girl, waited eight years before she conceived." (Interview, Katatura, January 1985)

One physician wondered about the connection between Depo-Provera and cervical cancer because he believed the incidence of cervical cancer to be particularly high in the north. (Interview, Walvis Bay, June 1985). Without careful investigation and monitoring of patients, however, any connection must remain speculative. In Walvis Bay, where Depo-Provera has been in use since the early 1970s, it was reported that rates of cervical cancer and breast cancer were both high (Interview, Walvis Bay, June

1985), but again only careful monitoring could demonstrate the connections. The association of Depo-Provera with cancer is well established, however, and the possible widespread incidence of cancer needs further investigation. It was difficult to check reports of high cancer rates in the political climate that existed during the period of research.

There has been much debate about Depo-Provera. It is argued that in some circumstances Depo-Provera is less risky than other contraception and that all contraceptives carry some dangers. Its use in Namibia, however, without public discussion, without consultation or even permission from the women receiving such injections constitutes a violation of human rights and not a justifiable family planning program in the interests of black Namibian women. Depo-Provera itself is not at issue here, though the use of Depo-Provera is problematic as has been indicated; at issue is the way in which the family planning program is conducted. The problem with Depo-Provera is that birth control by injections means control by medical personnel, not by the patient; once the injection is given the patient can do nothing until the effects wear off, which may take from six to eighteen months, and in rare cases several years.

It is worth noting that people who have tried to criticize the government's family planning policy have not found their task easy. The issue has become so sensitive in Namibia that anyone who dares to interfere with Depo-Provera stands accused of agitating against the state (Kazombaue 1987). Barbara Brown's comments about the indiscriminate use of Depo-Provera in Botswana are relevant here: "Using such a drug could backfire on the whole family planning program, jeopardizing its success. If some women suffer from one family planning method others might decide to oppose all." (Brown 1980)

Teenage Pregnancies

Teenagers are a specific group targeted by Depo-Provera campaigns because of the high rate of pregnancy among girls. The problem of teenage pregnancies illustrates the way in which the breakdown of the family and of social reproduction puts young girls at risk. The *Windhoek Observer* (November 11, 1987) carried an article about a motion tabled in the National Assembly to legalize abortion. A large part of this article was devoted to the high incidence of teenage pregnancies in Namibia. "A doctor at the State Hospital said that of the 4,000 deliveries in Windhoek each year, between 10 and 20 percent were from teenage mothers. About 20,000 babies are born in hospitals in the country each year and, although no statistics are available, it is strongly suspected that the percentage of teenage deliveries is about the same as at the Windhoek hospitals." Also reported was an extremely high dropout rate from schools in the areas of Rehoboth and Namaland, as a result of teenage pregnancies. A social worker reported that as many as twenty girls a year were forced to leave one school in Rehoboth over the last two years. "None of the authorities concerned were able to give figures," however.

> This reporter had the distinct impression that these figures were unavailable because such cases are removed from the ambit of schools as quickly and as discreetly as possible. School rules state that a girl must leave school immediately it is confirmed that she is pregnant. Girls then become the sole responsibility of the parents and the school has nothing more to do with her except that it may arrange for her to sit privately for matric examinations. Only in rare cases is any effort made by the schools to provide educational help. (*Windhoek Observer* November 11, 1987)

Hospital authorities also stated that backstreet abortions and occasionally infanticide were common ways of dealing with such pregnancies. It is possible legally to terminate pregnancies if girls are under sixteen years old, because the pregnancy is officially regarded as the result of statutory rape, but abortions are rarely done in Namibia, although hospitals in Cape Town do them in these circumstances. The newspaper article also reported that the hospital authorities called for state action in promoting contraception: "Hospital authorities in Windhoek said that they felt more should be done by the state to promote contraception, and one doctor said that this would be a far better way of fighting the overpopulation problem." (*Windhoek Observer* November 11, 1987)

In fact the hospital authorities are already giving considerable attention to the problem, and so are state-run clinics. There is only one clinic in Katatura and six nurses for a population of 37,000. One of the primary functions of this clinic is to give contraceptive injections, and women in Katatura have become wary of clinic staff making home visits. One informant reported that women hide and pretend to be out when they see clinic nurses for fear they might be coerced into having more Depo-Provera injections (Interview, Windhoek, October 1983). The following exchange is taken from an interview with one of the nurses working at the Katatura clinic in January 1985:

> *Question*: Can you tell me something about the contraceptive injections you are giving in the clinic?
> *Nurse*: Well, we are giving injections of Depo-Provera, you know.
> *Question*: What dosages are you giving?
> *Nurse*: We usually give 450 ml doses.
> *Question*: I've heard that contraceptive injections are given in the clinic to very young girls, even as young as thirteen or fourteen. Is this true?
> *Nurse*: Yes. We can't always tell how old girls are, you know. But we don't give them Depo-Provera, only Nur Esterate, in doses of 200 ml.
> *Question*: Do you give them injections without their parents' consent?
> *Nurse*: Yes. But if their parents complain then we don't give them a second injection, after the first.

This informant confirms that parents' complained of finding out that their daughters had been given contraceptive injections only when they returned from the clinic with a card stating so.

Giving contraceptive injections to young girls is a particularly disturbing practice, and the role of Katatura clinic is central to its continuation. There has been no organized public information campaign about the possible long-term consequences of hormonal therapies in terms that would make informed consent meaningful. Not surprisingly many uninformed but anxious parents are party to the practice. To protect their daughters from an early pregnancy which will, they know, add to the burdens of the whole family, as well as interrupt their education, and perhaps put an end to education altogether, mothers take their girls to the clinic. One mother declared frankly: "All my girls are getting Depo-Provera injections regularly. If they get pregnant that's a big problem and it's my duty to see that they don't." (Interview, Katatura, February 1985)

The social worker acting as interpreter on this occasion pointed out to me a young girl staying in this same house; her parents had beaten her, shaved off her hair, and turned her out of their house in disgrace when she became pregnant. Although the woman I had interviewed helped this young girl, she felt that the parents had been irresponsible in not taking her to the clinic for contraceptive injections.

Some teachers see contraceptive injections as the answer to schoolgirl pregnancy, and a school principal in the north suggested that this would be the way to deal with the problem in his school (Interview 1983). Another school principal in Katatura tried to coerce girls taking the matriculation examination into having contraceptive injections, threatening that they would not be entered for the exam if they refused (Interview with physician, Windhoek, February 1985).

In 1987 contraceptive injections began to be provided in Namibian secondary schools, according to Elago and Kazombaue (1988, p. 202):

> The government has introduced a program of family planning in secondary schools. Girls of menstruating age are injected with Depo-Provera in order to reduce teenage pregnancies in school. This program contradicts the Children's Act which is supposed to protect girls under 16 years of age to get involved [sic] in sexual activities. The moral implication this program has on the Namibian society is completely ignored. The young people are

encouraged to become sexually active at a tender age of 13 years; they are exposed to venereal diseases which result in low esteem. They see themselves as sex objects and many times young girls treated with Depo-Provera become prostitutes.

The costs of teenage pregnancy are high and some measures are urgently needed to protect young girls from early pregnancy. Parents are desperate. A physician in Windhoek spoke of fathers taking their daughters, sometimes as young as thirteen or fourteen, to private physicians for Depo-Provera injections: "They do this even when the girl doesn't have a boyfriend in order to protect their investment in higher education." (Interview, Katatura, October 1983)

In Walvis Bay, parents in the township of Narraville were so concerned about the high rate of teenage pregnancy that they called a parent-teacher meeting at the high school; they decided to ask the local hospital to send a nurse to the school so that girls could be given Depo-Provera injections (Interview, Walvis Bay, June 1985). Social conditions in Narraville also contribute to the problem, however; measures to reduce overcrowding might alleviate the situation. A Catholic priest commented wryly, "Twenty-five people sleeping in one house; someone's sure to get pregnant!" (Interview, Walvis Bay, June 1985).

Moreover, poverty in Walvis Bay is such that prostitution is a major source of income for many young girls. The same priest reported that girls told him, "I only sell my body because I'm hungry." (Interview, Walvis Bay, June 1985) Since the collapse of the fishing industry and the closure of the fish factories, unemployment in Walvis Bay has been constantly increasing and the overcrowded conditions in the townships of Narraville and Kuisebmond steadily worsen. Meanwhile houses in the white residential area stand empty.

Without full information parents cannot possibly be expected to make informed judgments about their daughters' welfare, and the lack of any public discussion has put parents in an immensely difficult situation. Some information about potential hazards of hormonal injections has recently penetrated the public media, however. In an article published in *The Namibian* (April 18, 1986), Nashilongo Elago noted the violence that is practiced on "young schoolgirls who are placed on this drug without the consent of parents." This article opened up discussion on a difficult subject.

In the north, Ovambo people traditionally attach great stigma to illegitimacy. Unmarried mothers may be unable to find a husband once they have given birth and will, in addition, be unable to continue their education at school. The civil war brought severe social dislocation in the north, accompanied by the disintegration of family and community controls, which were already eroded by the absence of men who migrated to the south as workers. Rates of illegitimacy are already very high. A church pastor reported that a girl living in his house was pregnant for the second time and that her situation was now desperate (Interview, Oniipa, January 1985).

A further element compounding the problem is the way in which middle-class professional men (teachers, administrators, police, and army) use their newfound wealth to bribe young women to give sexual favors. Such exploitative male/female relations within the black community are a manifestation of the triple oppression of class, race, and gender. The militarization of the northern territories of Ovambo, Kavango, and Caprivi forced many black women into prostitution. Many others are brutally assaulted and raped by soldiers of the South African Defense Force, both black and white. In war situations, black women are the particular victims of male aggression, their dehumanization and brutalization the most savage of all the manifestations of triple oppression (Brownmiller 1975; Enloe 1983). In a country in which poverty is widespread, the exploitation of women in the black working class takes place at the level of sexuality. Free availability of contraceptive injections, however safe or unsafe, compounds the exploitation.

The problem of teenage pregnancies in Namibia is undeniable, but is forcing the girls to have contraceptive injections the solution, or is sex education for girls and boys a better way to solve the problem? At the time of this research, there was no sex education in Namibian schools. This lack of information puts young girls at risk for hormonal injections, and it absolves men from reponsibility. The result is that pregnancy prevention, rather than the transformation of male/female relationships, is proposed. Some parents and pastors also argue that easy protection against pregnancy directly encourages promiscuity.

Sterilization

Health personnel have abused other forms of medical intervention such as the insertion of intrauterine devices and operations for sterilization and hysterectomy without permission or after the use of bullying and blackmailing techniques of persuasion.

Physicians and nurses in the refugee camps in Zambia and Angola discovered evidence of sterilizations carried out in hospitals in Kavango and Ovamboland, without the knowledge of the women concerned. Frieda Williams (1982) mentions such sterilizations. Airah Shikwambi, a Namibian health worker who worked in exile with the People's Liberation Army of Namibia, told an international seminar on Namibian health in 1982 that a number of women in the SWAPO refugee camps were sterilized when Namibian hospital personnel combined Caesarean sections with tubal resections without informing these women.

Many of the nurses interviewed reported that sterilizations in the course of Caesarean births, by means of cutting or tying the fallopian tubes, are common in Katatura Hospital; they added that Caesarean operations are performed frequently, if labor is at all protracted, often quite unnecessarily. When patients are reluctant to give permission for Cesarian sections they are panicked into doing so by suggestions that their lives are in danger (Interview, February 1985). Women from the north who wish to consult their husbands are bullied to take the decision alone when their husbands are working at some distance as migrant laborers or have remained in the north. At least one marriage in Ovamboland came to an end because the wife was sterilized in this way without her husband's permission during the course of Caesarean surgery: the angry husband promptly divorced the wife who could produce no more children.

SWAPO women confirmed reports of sterilizations in interviews. Both patients and nursing staff said that sterilizations in the guise of "a little biopsy" or "a little operation" are widespread throughout Namibia. What frequently happens is that, in the course of other surgery, such as the removal of cysts and tumors, physicians perform hysterectomies or cut and tie the woman's fallopian tubes. A nurse related the following story:

> A woman who had been infertile for a long time came into hospital. She signed permission for what she understood to be a small operation for the removal of a polypus from her vaginal passage, enabling her to have children. She later discovered that they had removed the whole uterus. Can you imagine how she felt? (Interview, November 1983)

Patients may consent to surgery without any idea of what is involved. Many patients are not able to read at all and depend on the nurse or physician to explain what the form means. Sterilizations also occur and health personnel press women to give their permission.

Even a standard dilatation and curettage can lead to a hysterectomy. A teacher, interviewed in 1985, miscarried her first child: in the course of the dilatation and curettage usual in these circumstances, she was given a hysterectomy, with no consultation and without her permission. Patients suffering from ectopic pregnancies may also be subjected to insensitive surgery that ensures they will never become pregnant again. Although it is possible to remove the embryo and repair any damage to the fallopian tubes, it is common practice in Namibia to simply cut the tube, thus making it easier for the surgeon to remove the embryo, at the expense of the patient's fertility. There is a high incidence of such pregnancies in Namibia, but the cause is not known.

A physician interviewed in one of the northern hospitals spoke about a patient sent to Windhoek for minor surgery, involving the removal of a small tumor of the uterus:

> I remember this woman very well because she was so distressed. She had never had a child, so she was blaming me for what happened. While she was in Windhoek they removed her whole uterus, without her permission, and

without any discussion, either before surgery or afterwards. They gave her no explanation at all. What is more we have never had any report on this case from Windhoek. However, I must tell you this is by no means unusual. This woman is only one case among many and I remember her only because she made so much fuss when she came back, and because she blames the whole disaster on me. But in the present situation we are helpless to do very much for such patients. (Interview, January 1985)

Nurses in Katatura Hospital maintain that hysterectomies are often performed quite unnecessarily, sometimes due to careless diagnosis:

I remember a woman who came into the ward with abdominal pain and was recommended for a hysterectomy. Fortunately, one of the nurses warned her to consult a private doctor before giving permission. She followed this advice, and the private doctor diagnosed minor infection and gave her antibiotics: the infection cleared up quite quickly and she didn't need surgery at all. (Interview with nurse from Katatura Hospital, October 1983)

Perhaps the worst case of careless diagnosis was that of a girl who was operated on for cysts. "When they opened her up they found that she was in fact pregnant. They removed the fetus and hushed up the whole matter. The girl was never told the true circumstances." (Interview with nurse from Katatura Hospital, January 1985)

Some nurses are callous in the treatment of women patients, as the experience of one woman patient reveals. She was surprised to find that the scar for her appendix operation was running vertically down her abdomen: "You think we've taken out your womb, don't you," said the nurse. She has not become pregnant since and fears they may have done just that.

Though most of my information relates to Katatura, such practices occur at other hospitals as well. Catholic nursing sisters at Rundu and Grootfontein refused to assist at surgical operations because of the irresponsible surgery they had witnessed (Interview with Catholic priest, Walvis Bay, 1985). Medical personnel performed sterilizations, both during the course of other surgery and as a "voluntary" measure for preventing births, in the hospital for black patients at Walvis Bay. An informant told me:

> Women are being forced into agreeing to sterilizations, particularly women from the Topnaar community who are admitted to hospital for delivery and considered to have too many children. One woman was told that she would not be allowed to go home unless she agreed to sterilization. (Interview, Walvis Bay, 1985)

In societies that place a high value on fertility, sterilization is a particularly serious matter and, even in situations that give good grounds for sterilization, there is reason for caution. One woman interviewed in Katatura was sterilized after she had given birth to five children by different fathers. Later she married and her marriage might have been happy but for her inability to have children, which was considered unforgivable. The man's family encouraged him to find new girlfriends, and he was constantly leaving his wife, returning, and then lapsing again. Sterilization did not solve her problems, it created new ones.

It is important to remember that some women elect sterilization. During a group discussion in Katatura, one woman spoke clearly about her decision to be sterilized in the near future. The importance of discussion and personal choice became clear as all of the women present talked about this decision and its implications. There is a difference between the dissemination of information, discussion, and personal decision making about family planning and sterilization, on the one hand, and the authoritarian program of population control in operation in Namibia before independence, on the other hand.

Intrauterine Devices

Interference with women's fertility during the course of surgery is widespread and can occur in a number of ways. Both patients and nurses in Katatura reported the insertion of Lippes Loop and Copper T intrauterine devices (IUDs) after dilatation and curettage. Although IUDs are not generally available and are expensive (they cost thirty-two rand in 1985), some physicians insert these devices without the permission or even knowledge of the patient, while she is under anesthetic. A nurse interviewed in 1984 told the following story:

> In 1980 I was suffering from very heavy menstrual bleeding and I went into the Katatura Hospital where I had a D and C [dilatation and curettage]. Several months later I had very bad pains in the abdominal region, so I went to my doctor. He told me that it was my IUD that was causing the trouble and that I had an infection. I was astonished. "What IUD?" I asked. He showed me the Copper T that he removed. I can only believe that it was inserted while I was in hospital, as I never had such a device. (Interview, London, July 1984)

This informant spoke both Afrikaans and English fluently and there could have been no communication problems. Moreover, she was a nurse and would have fully understood any explanation given to her. In fact she was told nothing. Another woman went to her physician because of a vaginal infection. She was surprised to find that the cause was a Lippes Loop, presumably inserted during a dilatation and curettage performed two years earlier (Interview, January 1985).

A former matron of Katatura Hospital interviewed in 1984 stated that African women did not like IUDs and that she estimated that there were no more than half a dozen of them in the whole of Katatura. The illegal insertion of IUDs, which are not even available in the family planning clinic in Katatura, constitutes one of the contradictions of the family planning campaign in Namibia. Implementation of population control policies is not consistent throughout Namibia and sometimes specific practices appear to occur as the result of individual initiatives by some physicians.

The Problem of Infertility

Although the illegal government of Namibia considered overpopulation to be a major threat, childlessness is the problem that worries many Namibian women. Medical authorities recognize three categories of childlessness: infertility, pregnancy loss, and child loss (Bergstrom 1981; WHO 1978). In Namibia, high infant and child mortality rates result in substantial child loss in the black communities. There is also considerable pregnancy loss: malaria, which is known to contribute to pregnancy loss, is still endemic, and puerperal fever is on the increase, although it ceased to be a notifiable disease in 1978 (Andersson 1984). According to recent reports, also on the increase is brucellosis, a disease that is contracted through contact with cattle and their carcasses or by drinking infected milk, which may lead to infertility (Andersson 1984). In the light of this report, a story related by a journalist who traveled in Kaokoland is of interest. Women asked him if he could give them an injection. Further enquiries revealed that they were infertile and hoped that an injection would cure them. He was told that infertility was widespread in the area and that women frequently suffered spontaneous abortions. (Interview, Windhoek, January 1985) Is it possible that women in this cattle-keeping community were suffering from brucellosis?

In addition, infertility caused by blockage of the fallopian tubes as a consequence of gonorrhea is a problem that needs investigation. Andersson (1984) reported a "dramatic increase in syphilis and particularly gonorrhea" in 1978. One of the nurses interviewed in January 1985 considered that infertility was simply not taken seriously:

> I knew a young woman who came into hospital to be operated on for cysts on the uterus. During the operation they found a blockage of the fallopian tubes and cleared it. She had been asking for help for some years and the doctor only gave her tablets, so it was only by accident that her infertility was cured. (Interview, Windhoek, 1985)

The problem of infertility worries many black Namibian women, but the medical services give it scant attention; in fact they make it difficult for women to obtain treatment. Couples receive treatment at the fertility clinics in Katatura only if they can produce a marriage certificate from a magistrate's court. Those married in a traditional ceremony do not qualify. Moreover, women who already have children are not treated at the clinic, even though it may be important to them to have more children—with a new husband, for example (Interview with physician, Windhoek, February 1985).

Conclusions

It is difficult to know why South Africa considered its population control policies to be appropriate for Namibia. One explanation is that South Africa consistently treated Namibia as if it were a province of South Africa, rather than a mandated territory; it ignored the inappropriateness of its population control policies because it has failed to acknowledge that conditions in Namibia are totally different from those prevailing in South Africa. An independent Namibia needs to reconsider these policies carefully.

What should be done about the provision of Depo-Provera?

What are the implications of the research findings? One option is to ban Depo-Provera. Zimbabwe banned this injectable hormone immediately after independence but has since reintroduced it as a result of popular demand for a wider range of contraceptive choices. IUDs and contraceptive pills are arguably as risky as Depo-Provera: IUDs can cause pelvic inflammatory disease, which is sometimes fatal; oral contraceptives, especially some high estrogen Pills, may have short-term and long-term side effects. If Depo-Provera continues to be available, physicians should give women thorough medical check-ups and monitor their progress, noting the side effects they experience. This practice is consonant with the manufacturer's recommendations. (Upjohn has a subsidiary plant in Johannesburg.)

The main form of contraception available in the refugee camps in Zambia and Angola was the contraceptive Pill. Namibian women returning from the camps are likely to demand continued access to oral contraception at clinics and hospitals. At the time of research, there was very little choice available to women in the black townships: Depo-Provera was the primary contraceptive method. A wider choice of contraceptives and the administration of all contraception on a more controlled basis would seem sensible. The Depo-Provera dosage administered in Katatura is exceptionally high. It would seem advisable to return to the standard dosage of 150 milliliters as recommended by the manufacturer. In addition, the use of Net-Oen for young girls should be considered carefully.

Above all family planning should be integrated into programs concerned with the overall health of women and their children. One obstacle to this ideal is the lack of trained staff.

What are the effects of Depo-Provera on the Namibian population?

Depo-Provera has been in use in Namibia for more than fifteen years. In Walvis Bay it has been in use for nearly twenty years. We do not know the long-term effects of Depo-Provera. The incidence of breast cancer and cervical cancer are reportedly high in Walvis Bay, but there is no systematic monitoring of women's health. Similarly, cervical cancer is reportedly widespread in northern Namibia, but again there is no systematic monitoring of the situation: indeed, the shortage of medical personnel in northern Namibia has reduced medical services to a minimum.

A campaign to give women Papanicolaou smear tests throughout Namibia would be one way of taking immediate action; it could save many women's lives. Even if there is no correlation between Depo-Provera and cervical cancer, this is a basic health service that could be provided.

Careful monitoring of women who have used Depo-Provera over a long period of time would seem advisable, especially women who are now trying to become pregnant. If Depo-Provera does result in infertility, then it is not suitable for women who have not had children and must be reserved for older women who have completed their families, as in Zimbabwe.

The importance of other contraceptive methods

The incidence of AIDS in Namibia is presently very low, but it is very high in Zambia and Zaire, and it is likely to rise in Namibia and become a matter of serious concern. A campaign to promote the use of condoms would be doubly valuable: it would reduce the risk of AIDS and other sexually transmitted diseases. It would also shift some of the responsibility for pregnancy prevention to men; at present, women bear the entire burden. There is no sex education in schools at the moment, and this is a matter of some urgency for the health of Namibians.

What about abortion?

Abortion is illegal in Namibia and South Africa. In 1987 the Namibian press reported that the Department of Health was discussing the legalization of abortion. As might be expected, there was an immediate outcry against this proposal. It seems unlikely that independent Namibia will provide abortion on demand. Strong religious feeling, which has always militated against this provision, will not change with independence. In 1986 the black Lutheran Church discussed both abortion and contraception. It decided that the use of contraception was a matter for individual conscience, but that the termination of pregnancy was not in accord with Christian teaching and could not be condoned.

Women still resort to illegal abortions, however, and the wards in Katatura Hospital, for example, are filled with women suffering from infections as a result of such abortions. It is important for the government of independent Namibia to consider ways of dealing with this situation. Women are desperate because they cannot feed the children they already have: a system of child support that provides some basic income for all children would perhaps encourage women to have their babies, rather than risk abortion.

Infertility

At present the health services accord little priority to women who are childless, even though this is a serious problem for many women because children are central to their identity and status. The puppet government emphasized overpopulation and made no attempt to investigate the extent of infertility. A surprising number of women interviewed had never had a child or had had only one child. A journalist reported that during a visit to Kaokoland women asked him for injections to cure infertility.

The infertility clinic in Katatura is not very sympathetic to the cultural background of patients, and it is difficult for black women to get satisfactory treatment for their infertility. Perhaps the independent government could remedy this. The lack of trained staff will be a problem.

Primary health care

Primary health care in rural areas would do much to reduce the high rates of sexually transmitted diseases, tuberculosis, and other infections responsible for infertility. Primary health care would also help reduce the high rates of maternal deaths. It is widely recognized that the independent government urgently needs a network of primary health care centers to replace the urban-based system presently in operation, which is geared to the needs of the white population. At Otjimbingwe, the people have already taken matters into their own hands and have set up a people's clinic to compensate for the inadequate health care existing in that community. Part of the system of primary health care will certainly focus on the needs of women and children, and it is likely that family planning will remain an important service. It is essential therefore to consider carefully the inadequacy of existing provision, both its stress on one form of risky contraception and its delivery of contraceptive advice.

Women need better information, a wider range of contraceptive choices, and to be listened to more sympathetically. Under the puppet regime, health care was delivered in an authoritarian manner. Because family planning is centrally important in every society, it is to be hoped that a full investigation of the population question in Namibia can and will take place in independent Namibia.

· 10 ·

Women, Children, and Health in Côte d'Ivoire

AGNÈS GUILLAUME*

IN AFRICAN SOCIETY, motherhood has for a long time dominated women's image. To acquire a social standing, women had to prove their fertility. Barren women were ill regarded and sometimes rejected by society (Locoh 1984), and some women sought compensation by fostering a child to give the appearance of motherhood.

Despite recent social changes, Ivorian women are still burdened with this prejudice. Women are of interest more because of their procreative than their productive capacities. Fertility does insure the renewal of the bloodline and the growth of the population, but women also contribute to daily survival inasmuch as they are responsible for maintaining the household and assuring the health

---

*Translated from French by Meredeth Turshen.

and education of children. Despite these responsibilities, women's economic and productive activities are not always recognized. Often classified as housewives, they are thought to be economically inactive. In this chapter, we analyze several censuses and surveys in order to comprehend the diversity of women's economic activities and to identify the real productivity of women's work.

Women sometimes find their worklives disrupted by the numerous children in their charge. The number of dependent children changes during the family's life cycle. Too many children constitute a brake on a woman's career, requiring her to remain at home; too few children constitute an obstacle if she depends on family labor, as for example in agricultural work. Women respond to these situations by distributing children to different family units. We report here on our study of child migration in Côte d'Ivoire and its economic and social consequences for women and children.

Women are in charge of family upkeep—food, health care, and children's education. How do they react when their children fall ill? What power do they have to decide on the care to be given? We address these questions in the final section of this chapter. Our response is based on research we carried out in various parts of Côte d'Ivoire, notably the southwest in 1989 and the southeast in 1986. These sociodemographic studies focused on the living conditions of women and children and on health and reproduction. We took an anthropological approach to health problems and interviewed traditional healers. This research is not representative of all women in the country but does illustrate their behavior when seeking health care in certain socioeconomic contexts.

Women Adapt Their Economic Activity to the Crisis

After a long period of remarkable growth from 1964 to 1977 (Dumont 1990, 23), Côte d'Ivoire experienced an economic crisis linked in part to the dramatic fall in the prices of coffee and cocoa, the primary products that are the main supports of the Ivorian economy. This crisis and the implementation from 1981 of structural adjustment policies have had serious economic repercussions; some of the main consequences are budgetary restrictions especially in the nonproductive health and education sectors, the elimination of nationalized enterprises, layoffs, cuts in wages and salaries, and the inability of planters to pay laborers.

In these circumstances, economic activity takes on an underground character and becomes difficult to identify. The informal sector expands as people engage in numerous activities and many petty occupations. Initially, these activities supported a marginal population of young people and school dropouts; in times of crisis they tend to expand and become fulltime occupations or parttime complements to other work. Women are also caught up in these informal activities.

Most socioeconomic studies ask some questions about occupation, but the criteria used to define employment vary. Some examples are: main activity, highest earning work, the job to which most time is devoted, the most productive work. The results vary depending on the number of responses accepted for each person. If the survey encodes one activity only, women generally give their occupation as housewife because, whatever their age, their place of residence, and their socieconomic milieu, all women do domestic work and raise children. As a result they are mistakenly considered to be inactive in terms of their employment status, and they are classified together with retired persons, invalids, and children.

The 1975 Ivorian population census classified 46.2 percent of women aged 15 to 59 as active and 49 percent as housewives. In 1978, a multi-round survey that used the technique of repeated visits over time and paid particular attention to women's employment (Oudin 1984) found 66.4 percent of women active and only 29.8 percent housewives, now defined as "women who do nothing other than unpaid housework" (Direction de la Statistique 1982). The importance of women's work emerges from the second set of figures. Fewer than one-third are exclusively housewives, while the active women do housework in addition to other work. If employment figures counted housework as an occupation, the rate of women's employment would approach that of men's.

Productivity gains linked to the activity of housewives are not easily or directly measurable, but their economic consequences are not negligible. By feeding and maintaining the family, women ensure the survival of its productive forces, and by their fertility they guarantee the reproduction of the labor force.

Fertility in Côte d'Ivoire remains high, about seven children per woman (Direction de la Statistique 1984). This large number of dependent children limits women's employment possibilities outside the home, especially in urban areas where the social cohesion is weakening and childcare by members of the extended family less available. No public or private daycare system exists to relieve women of this task. Also, because there are not enough places in school to accommodate all children, education begins at a later age and young children are at home in their mothers' care for a longer period. The practice of sending children away is a means of coping with an inadequate system.

Economically active women are self-employed or work in agriculture, trade, handicrafts, and as domestics; these occupations can be combined with housework. Few women are salaried because they lack the education and qualifications necessary for many types of paid employment.

Women's Work in Rural and Urban Areas

Faced with economic difficulties and, in some cases, with marital instability (about 10 percent of women in our study population are separated or divorced), women diversify their activities in order to meet their needs and acquire financial autonomy. Rare are those women who work fulltime in a single occupation.

Agricultural work is usually divided along gender lines; the allocation and number of tasks vary by region and by type of farm. Women have always participated in food production; in some areas they virtually monopolize this work. The development of the plantation economy and the introduction of cash crops brought about a redistribution of work roles in families that use family labor only.

Southeastern Côte d'Ivoire is one of the oldest sites of the plantation economy. Here women work in both sectors but they control food production while men control cash crops. Subsistence production furnishes 98 percent of the food consumed in the home.

In addition, women process food crops—for example, they turn manioc into semolina (*l'attiéké*) and palm nuts into palm oil. Raw and processed foods are either consumed at home or traded on the local market or in Abidjan; 65 percent of women sell their produce at least once a week. Women also resell such products as spices and dried fish which they purchase elsewhere (Guillaume 1988).

In the southwest the plantation economy has been expanding in the last ten years; here men participate more often in food production, although some tasks such as sowing and weeding are still women's work. Women also work in cash crops, especially when the planter who heads the household to which the women belong is unable to hire laborers. Women draw hardly any profit from their participation in the plantation economy both because they lose some of the income obtained from the production and sale of food and because men control the distribution of coffee and cocoa earnings (Guillaume and Diahou 1989).

Women's activities are very diverse in rural areas. As cultivators, they supervise all food production and work in cash cropping; as artisans, they process food; and as traders, they sell their produce. Clearly, all this work is on top of their housekeeping, which includes fetching water and firewood, preparing meals, and caring for children. Is women's work the same in urban areas?

Women's work is more varied in cities because the urban economy in more diverse; like their rural sisters, urban women do many different things. The examples given here are of two groups of women, those who live in Sassandra, a coastal city of 10,000 inhabitants situated in the southwest, and those who live in the slums of Abidjan in precarious circumstances that oblige them to adopt special survival strategies.

In Sassandra, 26 percent of the women produce food, 29 percent process fish, and 22 percent are traders (Fiege 1985). Seven percent of women are service workers; they run small restaurants (called *maquis*) and bars, and they are commercial sex workers. Three percent work in the public sector, and 2 percent in crafts, dressmaking, and food processing. Ten percent of women are without work.

The Fanti people, originally from Ghana, run the local fishing business, an important activity in which there is a clear division of labor: men fish and women smoke the catch and sell it.

Eighty-four percent of women traders sell food; others sell clothing, jewelry, cosmetics, and soaps and other household cleaning products.

In Abidjan's shantytowns, trading is women's main activity. They sell a wide variety of products—fruit and vegetables, prepared food, spices, etc. Asked why they trade, 58 percent say that trading is a vocation or a necessity, 23 percent invoke the need for a second income, 9 percent say that they trade because it is readily accessible, and 7 percent claim that it is profitable. When they trade close to home, women are sometimes helped by family members (20 percent of all aid comes from this source). Even when the income is meager, women say that trading is one of the few occupations open to them.

This review of women's economic activity shows how aberrant it is to think that women are inactive and how necessary to understand better the real extent of their activities. Studies of time and work give a better measure of women's productivity and their allocation of time to different activities than do economic surveys. As to the types of activity, agriculture and trade are the refuges of undereducated and underqualified women who have no access to more skilled work. Women turn to trading because it requires only a small investment and few qualifications and because it guarantees a regular income, however meager. Trading also allows women to reconcile work and child care responsibilities.

When high levels of fertility constitute an obstacle to remunerative work, women respond by redistributing their children to various units of the family.

Child Rearing

The mobility of children in the family or clan is an institutionalized phenomenon in West Africa. The number of children a woman raises in the course of her life does not necessarily correspond to the number she bears. Depending on the period in the family cycle and women's activities, women may decide that they have too many or too few children. A balance is established by redistribution, which entails either placing the children in other units of the extended family or receiving related or unrelated children in one's own. The fact that some children are not raised by their biological mother should be seen in the context of societies in which the idea of "mother" includes the biological mother, her sisters, the daughters and sisters of her maternal uncles, and her co-wives.

The Basis of Child Exchange

Child exchange is grounded in the fact that children do not strictly belong to either their mother or their father but to their parents' clan and may be reared by other family members. The transfer of children takes various forms: the simple loan of a child, guardianship, adoption for a fixed period of time, and as collateral or payment for a debt. All these forms of placement entail the delegation of parental rights and reciprocal obligations between families. For example, among the Baoulé, young brides frequently receive a child when they leave their parental home to join their husbands; if the child is a girl, she in turn will give one of her children to her foster mother.

These gifts of children have not only a social importance in raising the status of the guardian and in reinforcing his or her links with the group of the child's origin, but also an economic impact because the children often contribute to the economic activities of the foster household, particularly to the foster mother's work. Currently, these transfers are no longer limited to the clan; it is now common to have recourse to nonfamily labor.

Child migration is found in varying degrees in different parts of Côte d'Ivoire. Families in both rural and urban areas exchange children. In Abidjan about 20 percent of children under the age of twenty do not live with their biological parents. In some rural areas the figure is higher; about 45 percent of children in the Akan area, which is in the southeast about 50 kilometers from Abidjan, do not live with their biological parents. The figure is about 20 percent in northern Côte d'Ivoire.

For a long time, the direction of child migration was from rural to urban areas; it is now reversed, largely due to high rates of

TABLE 1
Status of Children in Households

	% Biologial	% Fostered
Abidjan 1978[a]	81	19
Southeast 1985 (Akyé)[b]	55	45
East 1986 (Baoulé)[b]	54	46
North 1987 (Sénoufo, Malinke)[b]	79	21
Abidjan 1987 (depressed areas)		
Total (under 20 years old)	82	18
Washington[c]	72	28
Gobelet[c]	90	10
Zoé Bruno[c]	70	30
Vridi Canal[c]	72	28

[a]unmarried children under 15 years old
[b]unmarried children under 20 years old
[c]dependents under 25 years old

SOURCE: Guillaume and Diahou 1989

urban unemployment and the difficulties of absorption in the cities. Urban dwellers more and more often confide their children to relatives in rural areas where the problems of survival are less acute and where access to education is easier because classrooms are less overcrowded and school fees are lower. The story of Gaston illustrates these issues.

Gaston, 48 years old in 1979, had migrated from the southwest to Abidjan and found a salaried job as head metal worker in a scrap metal business (Vidal and Le Pape 1986, 43). In 1979, his household comprised himself, his wife, eight children, and a young female relative. In 1984, the firm went bankrupt and Gaston was laid off. For a year he looked for work. In 1985, his wife was selling bananas around the new Marcory market, which is five hundred yards from their home. The two oldest sons were no longer in their father's charge. Three children were sent away to school: one to Oundo in western Côte d'Ivoire, one to Bingerville which is eight miles from Abidjan, and one to Korhogo in northern

Côte d'Ivoire. Remaining were the two youngest and a girl of twenty-one who was in high school. The household had shrunk from eleven to five members.

Child migration allows women to modify the number of children in their charge in the course of their lives. If one takes the case of women of childbearing age in Akyé (southeastern Côte d'Ivoire), 17 percent of their biological children do not live with them, but 9 percent of the children they raise are fostered. The percentages among older women are probably even higher.

Children are fostered at a very young age, on average at five years old. This displacement often entails early weaning; the children who were five at the time of our study had been taken in at the age of nine months. In these cases, the woman is really a substitute mother who must train the child for years before he or she can be of use to the household. In our study population, children left their mothers later, at about age nine. The difference between the ages at which children are fostered in and fostered out depends on the reasons for their exchange and the strategies of the women who make the decisions. The different motives for child migration explain the varying degrees of the practice from one region to another.

The reasons are not everywhere identical for girls and boys, at least not in magnitude. Schooling is generally the main reason for migration, except in the shantytowns of Abidjan in which education accounts for only 12 percent of the reasons given. For young girls undereducation is the rule. Mona Etienne (1987, 77) explains the reasons for undereducation of girls confided to Baoulé women in towns:

> Women tend to educate boys but rarely girls. This behavior has nothing to do with stereotypes, although it is somewhat related to the traditional division of labor. Girls work besides older women and thereby contribute immediately to income-generating activities. Boys play hardly any productive role in urban areas, although they do work in rural areas. To educate a girl is to lose the benefit of her productive contribution; it is to risk one's investment because if the girl becomes pregnant, she will have to

abandon her studies at least provisionally and probably
definitively. The money spent will have been wasted.

TABLE 2
Sex of Children Fostered In and Out for Education
(percent of all reasons)

Area and Year	Fostered In		Fostered Out	
	Boys	Girls	Boys	Girls
Abidjan 1978			70	29
Southeast 1985	73	46	47	40
Southwest 1989[a]	57	39	55	45

[a]Guillaume and Vimard 1990

SOURCE: Guillaume and Diahou (1989)

Placement as domestic help is the second most important
reason for child migration; it answers a need for labor in the foster
family. Farm help makes good the absence of biological children
who are at school and household help lightens the workload of the
guardian and allows her to engage in other work such as trading
or a salaried job. Thirty-one percent of girls, but only 12 to 13
percent of boys, migrate for this reason. Women who foster girls
and put them to work in the household in effect confine them to
the stereotypic female role of homemaker.

The use of child labor now extends beyond grandparents,
uncles, and aunts to unrelated families. In northeastern Côte
d'Ivoire, networks of recruiters supply cheap child labor to Abidjan
families (Diop 1989). Children so placed are generally illiterate
girls, eight to fifteen years old, from very poor families. Their
parents are led to believe the girls will live with the recruiter, who
is usually a relative of someone in the village; but in reality the
recruiter is merely an intermediary. He or she places the children
with strangers who put them to work as domestics or in the
informal sector. This system is advantageous to adults. The family
that supplies the girl will receive cash or a gift from the recruiter

when the child returns to the village, usually three to five years later. The recruiter in turn is compensated by the family that receives the girl, and he or she also enjoys a certain prestige in the village for bringing in money. The urban family benefits from the cheap labor of a child from whom they can exact unlimited work. The children hope to better their situation, a hope in which they are often deceived. One may well ask whether there is any real advantage for children in this system of transfers.

Initially, children left their biological parents for another home in order to be educated and to benefit from a richer social environment. Transfers are positive when they enhance the child's chances of success and offer better schooling as, for example, when the children gain entree to useful social networks by fraternizing with people from their region who are already assimilated in the city and perhaps belong to the elite.

But such is not the case for all children and particularly not for girls. With the economic difficulties that most households currently experience, the care of children becomes more and more problematic and only those capable of productive work are welcomed. Migration helps perpetuate the undereducation of girls who are generally placed as housemaids; it closets them in domestic roles and denies them access to training. It appears to us that the only hope these girls have of upward social mobility is in marriage, in which case they will exchange their dependence on their tutor for dependence on a husband.

Particularly when it extends beyond the family, child migration handicaps the psychological development of the child. Cut off from their origins (they rarely visit their biological family), children adapt to urban life. They leave the village as children and return as adolescents with a different set of values. Migration is equally detrimental when it subjects children to early weaning and heavy workloads. There is reason to fear that networks of child recruiters will expand, enriching adults, and that this form of child rearing will become commercialized and perpetuate the exploitation of children.

Whatever the objective relations, foster mothers must care for these children as if they were biologically their own. In the final section, we examine the health care aspects of child rearing in detail. How do women respond to illness, and what authority do they have to act on decisions that have financial implications?

Health Care for Women and Children

The role of women in child rearing is primary. Women assume the daily tasks of childcare and are the first to notice when a child falls ill. What options do they have to restore a child's health?

Health care choices depend on the existence of a public health care system and a private alternative. In Côte d'Ivoire, as in many parts of Africa, women can select traditional or biomedical care.

Traditional health care consists of consultations with a traditional healer or the use of home remedies (traditional medicines or pharmaceuticals). Traditional healers, diviners, and prophets prescribe care that may include the use of plants, prayers, chants, sacrifices, and purification rites. In addition to giving treatment, they try to find the reasons for the illness and the agents responsible for its appearance (Guillaume and Rey 1988). The healing virtues of certain plants are well known and this information is passed from one generation of women to the next. Plants are used to treat all illnesses that do not require a causal explanation. Self-medication is common where there are village pharmacies and where pharmaceuticals are sold illegally in markets or hawked door-to-door by traders.

The government has constructed biomedical health care facilities—hospitals, dispensaries, and maternities—in various parts of Côte d'Ivoire, but their distribution is uneven. In the 1984 meeting of the *Etats Généraux de la Santé* (Ministère de la Santé 1984), the government's evaluation of the health care system was as follows:

> The development of health services really took off in 1977 when substantial investments were made; it reached its peak in 1978, only to fall off and decline until in 1982, it reached its lowest level.... The part of the budget allocated to health is constantly declining—from 16.8 percent in 1971 to 7.5 percent in 1984.... Health facilities are

generally old, in bad condition, and no longer correspond to current medical needs. Hospitals, in particular, suffer from a notorious lack of material in all services, in Abidjan and the interior of the country. By material we mean technical material, supplies and equipment. . . . Most of the (health care budget) is invested in Abidjan. . . . The ratio of hospital beds to population passed from 1:1,247 in 1949 to 1:867 in 1982, but the distribution between urban and rural areas is uneven, to the detriment of rural areas.

In terms of medical personnel, the situation is unsatisfactory. In 1982 there was one doctor for every 15,000 people, one nurse for every 3,000 people, and one midwife for every 10,000 people, and the personnel are unevenly distributed. "In the interior of the country, there are maternities without midwives, whereas in some cities there are twenty midwives in a maternity that delivers only one baby per day" (ibid.). In some urban health facilities the workload is so heavy that the personnel are rude and patients feel that they are poorly cared for.

This critique of health care in Côte d'Ivoire reveals a system in disarray. Government health care is free but it is not always accessible because of the lack of clinics, lack of supplies and equipment, lack of drugs, lack of personnel, or because personnel are not qualified. In face of this penury, women tend to assume costs that are normally borne by the public health system, for example, the costs of surgical supplies and medication. In addition, they have to shop for these items because the centers are supplied only twice per year and do not have sufficient stock to meet demand. These deficiencies do not encourage women to frequent health centers, especially those women who are not in the habit of attending clinics.

People are confronted with several health care systems, each with its advantages and disadvantages. What guides women in their choice of care for themselves and their children?

Reasons for choosing one or another type of health care are complex. Of course availability is determinant, but there are other considerations. Cultural constraints may dictate a precise line of conduct: for example, an illness considered "natural" is treated simply with home remedies or at a dispensary. If the illness is thought to be "induced," "the patient will systematically select a therapist and healer able to treat the cause and a dispensary to suppress the symptoms" (Guillaume and Rey 1988, 8). Economic restraints, lack of money or lack of time, also limit visits to biomedical health care centers, especially when clinics are far from home and the cost of transport must be added to the cost of medical supplies (described above). Family constraints, such as the number of children and proximity to parents (mothers have an important influence on the choice of therapies), also determine the type of care sought. What choices do women make?

Health Care Behavior

Women's choice of health care for themselves and their children varies according to whether they seek prenatal care, postnatal care, treatment for illness or for infertility.

In southwestern Côte d'Ivoire 42 percent of the children under five years in our study population were ill in 1988. Women's responses were varied: in almost half (49 percent) of the cases they took the children to biomedical facilities (dispensaries and hospitals); they chose traditional care in 32 percent of the cases; and in the remaining 19 percent they alternated between traditional and biomedical care, with biomedical care usually being the woman's first choice.

That one-third choose traditional care alone shows how common this practice is. In this category, women selected home remedies from the family medicine chest in 73 percent of the cases: clearly, home remedies are very important and have many advantages—low cost, few time constraints, no travel, and ready availability.

In childbirth, 61 percent of women in the southwest go to a hospital or maternity, and 35 percent remain at home to be looked after by the family. Women who give birth in a hospital are better followed during pregnancy (3.9 prenatal consultations) than women who give birth at home (1.5 visits). Nineteen percent of all women, however, receive no prenatal care, which they explain by saying that the health centers are too far away (70 percent), too expensive (15 percent), or too unfamiliar and inhabitual (8 percent). The first two explanations are interrelated because distance is linked to cost: travel requires an availability of time and money.

In southeastern Côte d'Ivoire, women's health care behavior is slightly different. To care for their children, far more women use biomedical services (68 percent) or a combination of biomedical and traditional care (24 percent). Only 8 percent use traditional treatment alone. Specific choices here as in other regions are linked to the type of illness. For example, when seeking help for infants suffering from what is called locally the "fontanelle sickness," women's behavior changes: 42 percent go to dispensaries, 31 percent seek a combination of biomedical and traditional care, and 27 percent use traditional treatment alone. The changed behavior is related directly to the specific illness: women consider depression or movement of the fontanelle (a membranous space between the cranial bones) "induced" rather than "natural" and they say openly, "Whites don't know how to treat that."

In terms of their own health, half of the women questioned in the southeast reported that they had been ill the previous year. In illness, 60 percent of women attend a dispensary; 27 percent seek a combination of biomedical and traditional care; and 5 percent use traditional treatment alone. For prenatal care, 65 percent of women attend a dispensary; 31 percent seek a combination of biomedical and traditional care; and 4 percent use traditional treatment alone. In contrast, in the case of an illness related to primary or secondary infertility, biomedical care accounts for only 43 percent of consultations, combined biomedical and traditional care account for 50 percent, and traditional care alone accounts for 7 percent. The difference in behavior is again linked to the type of illness. Women mention three causes of infertility: among those who have never been pregnant, infertility is thought to be incurable, an illness decreed by god, which exists from birth; among women who have conceived, infertility is thought to be related to sickness during the childbearing years; and the third explanation is witchcraft. In cases of infertility it is necessary both to determine the reasons for the condition which require sacrifices to abate it, and to treat the clinical signs by going to a dispensary or by using traditional remedies.

Women thus adopt a multitude of therapeutic behaviors, but are they really the decision makers?

Women appear to have more autonomy in deciding on health care for themselves than for their children. Although women alone assume the daily care of children, their husbands frequently intervene in decisions on children's health care. Men are responsible for 41 percent of the choices; women take sole responsibility 43 percent of the time. Men and women have slightly different notions of what constitutes adequate care. When women alone make the decisions, they choose traditional treatment in 59 percent of cases; men more frequently decide to consult biomedical facilities (58 percent of cases).

How are these decisions justified? Women are attracted to home remedies, the most traditional of therapies, for two reasons. First, they alone have this knowledge, which is usually inherited from their mothers; and second, this care is free (in 48 percent of cases) or affordable, which is important as they are not sufficiently financially autonomous. Men are usually financially responsible for health care (61 percent of costs borne by husbands).

Women are responsible for children's health but they are not entirely free to decide on the type of care because their husbands intervene. This dependent health care behavior appears to be related to their lack of autonomy, which is caused in part by their lack of financial independence and in part by their low levels of education. The lack of financial autonomy limits women's choices, and low levels of education hamper their ability to adopt new health care behavior easily.

Conclusion

Ivorian women, in cities and in the countryside, play central productive and reproductive roles in their families and in society generally. Because their productive roles are not always recognized (at least not in certain studies), there is a tendency to think of them only as housewives and therefore as economically inactive. In fact women's activities are many and varied. With the economic crisis, women have diversified their activities in order to increase their income and acquire some financial independence. Their housekeeping activities are combined with those of farming, handicrafts, or trading, or some combination of all three. The fact that the real value of women's work is not recognized is deleterious to their living standards and has a negative effect on their health and that of their children. Failure to recognize women's contribution also has an impact on the economy generally, which is badly planned when it excludes women. Women are often neglected in local development plans, and the result seems to be a perpetuation of their economic and social dependence on men.

Women's importance in society stems equally from their reproductive role: they insure the survival of the family and the continuity of the bloodline by their fertility, but they also ensure daily survival inasmuch as they are responsible for the upkeep of the home and for the feeding, education, and health care of children. Women who produce food in the rural areas practically guarantee the family's self-sufficiency.

With the economic crisis, living standards have declined, and the deterioration of material conditions has had negative effects on women and children's health. The adjustment policies implemented to improve the economic situation have also aggravated the health situation by draining the public health care system.

Better trained women would be able to acquire more autonomy, gain access to other economic sectors, and become more efficient in their current work. Higher qualifications depend on equal access to primary and secondary school for girls and boys and on women's access to vocational training. The exclusion of girls from the educational system is partly linked to a mentality that confines women and girls to housework and the home. Child migration, particularly in the context of recruitment networks, reinforces this mentality insofar as young girls are exploited as domestics.

Progress in women's access to education will have an impact on daily life, especially in the area of health care. If women's productive roles were recognized, girls would be integrated into the educational system. The increased productivity that would result would offer better living standards to women and their children. These changes could be brought about by women's participation in development plans.

· 11 ·

Gender, Power, and Risk of AIDS in Zaire[1]

BROOKE GRUNDFEST SCHOEPF,
WALU ENGUNDU, RUKARANGIRA
WA NKERA, PAYANZO NTSOMO,
AND CLAUDE SCHOEPF

AIDS, ACQUIRED IMMUNE deficiency syndrome, a new lethal communicable disease syndrome, has rapidly developed into a world-wide pandemic affecting some 140 countries, including forty-three in Africa. The human immune deficiency virus (HIV) which causes AIDS is transmitted from infected persons by sexual contact and blood, and from mother to fetus. In Central Africa, where infection occurs primarily as a result of heterosexual intercourse with an infected partner, women tend to predominate among both people testing positive for HIV and people with AIDS.[2]

This chapter presents ethnographic research conducted by the CONNAISSIDA Project in Zaire since February 1985; the project aims to develop a broad understanding of the spread of infection, the cultural construction of AIDS, and the impact of the syndrome on the population of Zaire's two largest cities. These are Kinshasa and Lubumbashi, with a combined total of more than four and one-half million people.

The methodological approach is related to a number of advances made in the study of continuity and change in African societies over the past two decades. Three of these are crucial. The first is the importance of understanding how the macrolevel political economy affects sociocultural dynamics at the microlevel—including the spread of disease and social response to epidemics. The condition of women, culturally constructed gender roles, and concepts of personhood are central to these processes, as are historical and contemporary relations between Africa and the West. The second is the attention to countercurrents of resistance to dominant ideologies and structures. Gender roles need not be static, and recent scholarship has brought to light many examples of women's struggles to change their condition. The third is the linkage between sectors of the economy often conceived as separate, for example, between formal and informal, traditional and modern, or rural and urban sectors. Such linkages are essential to understanding processes of sociocultural change, the political ecology of disease, and disease prevention. In this context, the condition of women is emblematic of the process of capital accumulation which drains resources away from the villages, upward to national ruling classes, and outward to world markets.

In Zaire, as elsewhere in Africa, heterosexual transmission accounts for the vast majority of HIV infections, and there are no special risk groups. With infection levels reported at 6 to 9 percent among sexually active urban adults in 1986 (N'Galy, Ryder, and Bila 1988), primary prevention involves convincing many among the general population to alter behaviors which are widely considered "normal" and "natural," but which nonetheless place people at risk for AIDS.

Although there is no evidence that Africans are more sexually active or more "promiscuous" than people elsewhere, several types of multiple partner relationships are culturally valued in various social milieus. Others, while not positively sanctioned, are condoned by some and practiced by many. There are also exclusively monogamous couples and celibate single people.

AIDS prevention is particularly complex, for it is subject to multiple cultural interpretations and resistance. Transmission is related to blood, semen, and vaginal secretions. In Central Africa these body substances are freighted with symbolic significance and cosmic importance. Moreover, sexual relationships and procreation are essential elements of what makes life worth living. Their performance is related to the personal identity and self-worth of women and men, and to health, wealth, and pleasure.

Our findings confirm studies conducted elsewhere, which indicate that increased knowledge is necessary but seldom sufficient to change behavior. By mid-1987 virtually all of the nearly six hundred adults and adolescents interviewed were aware that AIDS is a fatal disease transmitted by sexual relations and blood. Many also knew that unsterilized instruments could be dangerous and those who could afford to do so bought disposable syringes. Few, however, were aware of transmission from mother to fetus. Misconceptions were common and very few people had abandoned risky sexual behaviors. Most people had not heard of condoms or had heard of them but did not know what they were.

Some constraints to change are situated at the microlevel of social interaction, internalized cultural prescriptions, and individual psychodynamics. Other constraints are situated at the macrolevel of the wider social system and international political economy. The action research described here shows how these interpenetrating social forces act to constrain change.

Economic Crisis, Gender, and AIDS

Disease epidemics generally erupt in times of crisis and AIDS is no exception. Zaire, like most other sub-Saharan nations and much of the third world, is in the throes of economic turmoil. Propelled by declining terms of trade and burdensome debt service, the contradictions of distorted peripheral economies with rapid class-formation have created what appears to be a permanent, deepening crisis. Zaire's crisis began soon after a period of growth between 1968 and 1973, which saw increased dependency on copper and other mineral exports that had dominated the colonial economy from the

1920s. Capital-intensive public investments made with foreign loans created relatively few new jobs. In 1974, declining international copper prices sent government revenues plummeting while debt service payments came due. Dearth of investment in peasant production and transport infrastructure fueled the exodus to cities already crowded with unemployed. To these liabilities were added redistribution of internal economic resources from foreign owners to Zairians linked to the inner circle of political power. The management of these windfalls has been much criticized. A cumulative negative growth rate of 18 percent occurred over the next decade and prices rose 6,580 percent. Per capita incomes are ranked among the world's lowest (World Bank 1986). Many urban families eat only once a day and malnutrition is widespread.

Throughout the continent, poor women and children have experienced most severely the effects of structural adjustment policies and the deepening crisis. In Zaire, as elsewhere in the region, economic crisis and the structure of employment inherited from the colonial period contribute to the feminization of poverty and consequently to the spread of AIDS.

In the early colonial period, wage labor was reserved to men, who were paid below subsistence wages, while women were constrained to crop production and frequent childbearing. Women who escaped to the cities resorted to petty trade and services, including sex. Even after independence in 1960, few wage labor opportunities for women were created. Currently, Zaire's cities contain as many women as men. An estimated 40 to 60 percent of urban men are without waged employment. They and the majority of women who are without special job qualifications resort to informal sector occupations. These include petty trade, food preparation, market gardening, sewing, smuggling, and prostitution. As the crisis deepens, illegal home manufacturing of beer and alcohol is also returning.

Not surprisingly, young urban women constitute the major risk group for AIDS in Central Africa. Professional sex workers are at highest risk. More than 90 percent of poor prostitutes are reported to be infected in several cities of Central and East Africa. They are not the only women at risk, however. Many other types of multiple partner relationships, with varying degrees of social recognition and legitimacy, exist among people of all social classes and ethnic origin. Polygyny continues to be widespread and polyandry continues as a minor theme. Even socially recognized relationships may be of relatively brief duration, leading, as in the West, to what has been termed "serial polygyny." At least half of Kinshasa's youth have had sexual experience by age seventeen (Bertrand, Bakutuvwidi, Kinavwidi, and Balowa 1989), and the rising age of marriage provides time for experimentation with multiple partners. Young women may use their charms to obtain the perquisites of urban dress—shoes, handbags, jewelry, cosmetics, and stylish clothes—which neither wages nor trade provide. At Kinshasa's city hospital, 16.9 percent of female employees aged 20 to 29 years were HIV-positive in 1986.[3] The corresponding rate among men was 9.3 percent (N'Galy, Ryder, and Bila 1988).

Not all multiple partner relationships are entered on the basis of women's consent. While forcible rape appears to be extremely rare, sexual harassment of women is reported to be common. For example, school girls and students may be required to provide sex to teachers or see their grades suffer. Numerous women state that they are required to extend sexual services to employers as a condition of employment and promotion. Some husbands refuse to allow their wives to work for wages because of this. Their refusal renders vulnerable many women who might otherwise have been able to earn a living without resorting to sexual strategies upon finding themselves divorced or widowed.

Attention tends to focus on casual sex when high-risk behaviors are considered. Nevertheless several forms of stable multiple partnerships are linked to informal sector activities and may contribute to the spread of AIDS. For example, male long-distance traders are likely to have several wives or women with whom they live in relatively stable unions in towns along their routes. Wives and children provide the trader with an identity as a responsible adult with a reason for being in the town. Their houses shelter the man's activities from the prying eyes that follow hotel guests and also provide secure storage for goods. Wives make trading contacts and obtain permits using their local kinship and patron-client networks. They also may trade on their own account with goods or capital supplied by the visiting husband. Some of these wives are monogamous; others have two or more husbands.

Women traders are perceived by many men as universally promiscuous. Since they are able to command their own resources, their sexuality is beyond male control. Women who are not deterred by moral scruples can use sexual strategies to economic advantage. Some develop regular sexual relationships with officials to facilitate obtaining permits and fee waivers (Schoepf 1981; MacGaffey 1986). Some use casual sex instead of cash to meet travel and trading expenses along their routes or at ports of entry. Although windfall profits can enrich some who participate in irregular trade, the risks are high for those without political protection. In addition to these instrumental sexual relationships, trading journeys also offer opportunities for recreational sex and emotional or erotic adventures.

As economic conditions continue to worsen, sexual strategies that maximize returns become increasingly important. One result of the crisis at the macrolevel is to render the already crowded informal economic sector increasingly less profitable for many small operators. Moreover, many women who formerly could rely upon steady contributions from partners or from their extended families report that both sources are dwindling because they, too, are hard-pressed to make ends meet. Women often seek occasional partners, *pneus de rechange* or "spare tires," to meet immediate cash needs. Although no statistics exist, our observations indicate that multiple partner situations, particularly those involving various forms of sexual patron-client relationships, appear to be increasing as a result of the economic crisis.

The health consequences of multiple partner strategies, often serious in the past (Schoepf and Schoepf 1981), have become much more so over the past decade. It is the fact of multiple partners, rather than the type of relationship, however socially categorized and labelled, which puts people at risk. At the same time, since many people cannot limit their sexual relations to a single, infection-free, lifetime partner, correct and regular condom use offers the best protection currently available. Other CONNAIS-SIDA publications analyze gendered perceptions of AIDS and present the economic, sociocultural, and psychological constraints that render condom use difficult in the Zairian setting (Schoepf et al. 1988a; Schoepf and Schoepf 1988; Schoepf et al. 1988b; Rukarangira and Schoepf 1989; Schoepf 1988). Action research addresses some of these constraints.

Risk-Reduction Workshops

CONNAISSIDA's action research is based upon ethnographic and experiential training methods. Experiential training is a method for introducing directed cultural change in formal organizations such as business and government; for developing management, leadership, and decision-making skills; and for imparting new knowledge to adults in a wide variety of settings.

Our first workshops engaged women residents of a low-income community, with little or no literacy, in a problem-solving approach to risk reduction. The workshop design uses active learning methods, including role plays, simple posters, small group discussions, and structured group "processing" to demonstrate to participants their own ability to reduce their risk of AIDS. Didactic presentations are kept to a minimum. The workshop leaders (or trainers) do not give advice; instead, they promote the search for solutions appropriate to the participants' lifestyles. Because the exercises crystallize real-life experiences, cognitive learning is stimulated by the emotional impact of the situation. Processing participants' reactions to what they have just done, seen, and heard in a group sets up a social filter for the learning experience. Groups quickly develop their own subcultures with norms and values that reinforce the learning of new skills and knowledge.

Grounded in principles of group dynamics, experiential training begins with the principle that people already know a great deal about their situation. Group leaders assist people to develop a "critical consciousness" leading to cooperative social action and self-reliance (Freire 1978; Hope and Timmel 1985). Although some risk-reduction strategies, including individual counseling, tend to emphasize making high-risk individuals responsible, the training strategy aims to develop the participants' personal power. In this case, power is defined as the capacity to control risky situations.

The difference between responsibility and empowerment is more than semantic. In the case of women—especially sex workers who experience social stigma, feelings of powerlessness, and low self-worth—telling them how they should act is tantamount to blaming them for their predicament. Instead of focusing on behavior that cannot be altered under present circumstances, experiential training helps people to discover what they can do to make their situation somewhat better in the short term. Although the method concentrates on self-empowerment, it also can be used to initiate and sustain other types of socially transformative change. The need to increase feelings of personal competence and to minimize anxiety and guilt, with their resulting denial, blame-casting, and avoidance, was identified from data contributed not only by women with multiple partners but by others variously situated socially.

The first experiment was conducted with a network of fifteen sex workers.[4] The women report serving between five and forty clients per working week. They charge very low fees and have had recurrent bouts of sexually transmitted diseases. In July 1987, most recognized that their activities placed them at high risk for AIDS. With no other way to support themselves and their dependents, however, their attitudes included apathy, fatalism, and denial. By October 1987, their awareness of AIDS had grown, partly as a result of the national mass media campaign; their existential dilemma could no longer be denied. As the national campaign against AIDS became more visible, the women reported that neighbors had begun pointing hostilely at them as "disease distributors." The leader of the network asked CONNAISSIDA to provide the group with information on AIDS prevention. Their experience of stigma led them to request that the workshops be held somewhere other than their open yard. We were refused space in a local church and held the sessions in a private garden, situated some 500 yards from their homes. Four morning workshops were held in late October and early November. A few examples will illustrate the intervention method.

An initial role play serves as an ice-breaker. It portrays a male visitor who fails to recognize that the woman who welcomes him to her village is a chief. (The scene is adapted from a passage in

David Livingstone's [1857] diary relating his visit to a Lunda group in what is now Zambia, where women chiefs were common a century ago.) The women immediately saw the visitor's problem and laughed at him.[5] Participants were asked to describe what they had seen, heard, and felt. Generalizing about what they had just seen, they remarked that women's responsibilities often go unrecognized. Applying this insight to AIDS, they concluded that they must take care not to become infected because AIDS is fatal and others, including children, siblings, and elderly parents, depend upon them for support.

Other exercises show how HIV progressively attacks the body's defenses against disease. Role plays demonstrate transmission routes and social situations that involve risk. A dramatization of mother-infant transmission elicited strong emotional reactions such as: "Oh, the poor thing hasn't even begun to live and now he's dying of AIDS!"

AIDS prevention is addressed in a broader community health context, which helps to remove some of the stigma and guilt associated with sexual transmission. For example, we include ways to prevent malaria, as one means to reduce the need for blood transfusions among anemic children. Sterilization of needles and syringes also is addressed, since poor people cannot afford to purchase disposables for each injection. Although unsterilized instruments are probably not a major route of HIV transmission (N'Galy et al. 1988), this route has been widely publicized. Role playing helps women to check on hygienic standards in local dispensaries. The experience is empowering and will help to reduce risk of other iatrogenic infections.

An entire session is devoted to condoms, demystifying what is to most an unfamiliar, uncongenial, unnatural, unwanted foreign technology. The group consumes soft drinks together. A trainer produces a box of condoms and irreverently displays one on her forearm. The condoms are passed around and each participant rolls one over her empty soft drink bottle. Some break, giving rise to jokes which provide opportunities for further teaching. In the ensuing role play, a sex worker shows a reluctant client how to use a condom, using her powers of seduction to eroticize the situation and overcome his resistance. The women take home condoms to try before the next workshop during which they share their experiences with the trainers and the group.

When a local Protestant Mothers Club learned of our workshops for sex workers, they requested that we come to their church to hold workshops, which we did. In this group we began by exploring the wider health context and then took up sexual transmission. We added a role play to help wives persuade husbands to remain at home instead of accompanying their friends to bars where they buy beer and sexual adventures. The drama enacted by participants showed how male peer group pressures work to prevent behavioral change. (This role play has proved useful in all-male and mixed sex groups as well.) Participants decided that although married women are definitely subordinate within the household, the wife-and-mother role also provides some opportunities to cajole husbands into dialogue about the need for protecting parents and children. The workshops provided a forum in which to practice communication skills and to develop confidence in parrying male resistance.

The "condom seduction" was expertly performed by two volunteers: a grandmother who was formerly a professional sex worker acted the reluctant husband; a young sex worker who is a member of the congregation acted the cajoling wife. Their inclusion in the church group taught the research team that categorization of women in mutually exclusive social/sexual status pigeonholes such as "prostitutes," "mothers," or "church members," can be misleading and counterproductive. Negative value judgments and reluctance to be associated with stigmatized social categories hinder people from examining their behavior and making realistic risk assessments.

In fact, sexual relationships vary according to the circumstances in which women find themselves at different moments in their lives. Several divorced, abandoned, or widowed mothers and their children were receiving alms from the congregation. The Mothers Club president emphasized that dire poverty and lack of economic alternatives made it likely that such women would soon become sex workers. Former sex workers who had attempted to find other means of support also feared that they would be obliged to resume this high-risk occupation. Working with the two groups simultaneously reinforced our conviction that for many poor women prostitution is not a profession but merely a survival strategy resorted to when other strategies fail.

Evaluation

User-focused evaluation meetings held at three and nine months following the risk-reduction workshops sought to discover participants' reactions to the interventions. We asked what changes, if any, had been tried and sustained. At the end of three months, all but one of the sex-workers reported using condoms regularly, both those supplied without charge by the project and those purchased at the local pharmacy. The non-user reported that a genital ulcer made condom use painful, so we drove her to the hospital, as local dispensaries are without testing facilities. Client acceptance of condoms was reported high. Two women said that they had turned away men who refused condom protection. Their colleagues agreed that this was a wise practice but that sometimes they needed immediate cash and had no other clients waiting.

Knowledge of condom protection apparently raised the women's status among clients and community residents. Clients were surprised to discover that the women knew about the value of condoms for AIDS prevention. The women felt somewhat less threatened by neighbors. Participants said that they would like the government to provide regular health examinations and testing for HIV infection, so that they might be issued health cards, as had been the case formerly with syphilis and other treatable sexually transmitted diseases. They had not grasped the significance of AIDS's long latency period and the continuing risk of an almost certainly fatal infection. These make such procedures illusory as protective measures in the case of AIDS.

The training was perceived as valuable. Participants asked: "Can you teach us to do what you do so that we can inform our colleagues?" Following a practice session, the sex workers demonstrated the method to friends in the presence of an international site visit team. Their performances indicated that considerable knowledge about AIDS had been retained. Condoms were made available on a continuing basis and the participants were encouraged to share their knowledge and supplies with others.

At nine months post-intervention, however, sex worker participants reported that condom use had declined from "almost always" to "sometimes." Their confidence in condom protection had waned. Two women said that student clients had told them that the condoms we supplied were outdated. They wanted us to provide a more attractive product being distributed by a contraceptive Social Marketing Project, which had achieved remarkable success in the interim (Mivumbi 1988).[6] By June 1988, the marketed product's brand name "Prudence" had become synonymous with "condom" among university students.

More serious was the undermining of the sex workers' recently developed need to use condoms by student clients who had read or heard about the April 7, 1988, issue of *Paris Match*, which carried an interview with U.S. sex researcher Jonathan Kolodney. Kolodney was quoted saying that condoms provide incomplete protection from HIV infection. In Kinshasa, this was translated to mean that condoms are useless. The relatively high-status students, a credible source of information, told the sex workers: "No need to use those things!" and the women acted upon this incorrect advice, for they were not ready to lose these preferred clients. Student clients are highly regarded by these poor women, who were born in the interior and have had little or no formal primary education. A television appearance that same week by the Public Health Department's AIDS coordinator, who promoted condom protection, did not prevail over the authority imputed to the international news media. Like most poor and working class inhabitants of Kinshasa, these women do not own radios or have access to television on a regular basis (Houyoux et al. 1986). They could not remember having heard anything about AIDS from media sources during the three previous months, nor can they read newspapers or handbills. Apart from "SIDA," a record of advice set to music issued by the popular singer Luambo in May 1987, and the CONNAISSIDA workshops, the "sidewalk radio" (gossip network) was their principal source of AIDS information. That this incident occurred in a community where a bar owner and three of the sex workers who paid him in kind for the right to solicit clients in his establishment had recently died of AIDS is testimony to the influence of social status as a determinant of popular knowledge.

Since communication systems are social systems, the reception of information and the ability to act on information received are differentially distributed in hierarchical systems. Differential social power needs to be considered when designing prevention strategies. Popular and biomedical sentiment consider prostitutes as the major reservoir of AIDS as of other sexually transmited diseases in Africa, as in the West. Viewed from a different perspective, however, the poor sex workers are at higher risk than their student clients. The women serve between two hundred and fifty and one thousand clients annually, whereas the students use their services once or twice per month. Condoms are commonly perceived as offering protection for men against women. This stigmatizing gendered perception is involved in many women's refusal of condoms, as we discovered from interviews in many different settings. The young men's disparagement of condoms and the sex workers' acceptance of their authority increases the women's risk. It also underscores the need for activities that can effectively increase their sense of self-worth and over the long term lead to empowerment.

Empowerment is an issue for the churchwomen as well. One-third of sixty participants reported that their husbands utterly refused to consider using condoms or even to discuss the risks the couple might face. Some of these were older men; their wives believed they no longer sought extramarital sex. Some husbands known to have multiple partners were reported to have responded with anger and hostile threats. For example, one woman said that her spouse refused to give her the monthly housekeeping allowance, telling her to go out and hustle for it. Another third of participants reported that they had been able to open a dialogue, but that their husbands had persuaded them that their risks were negligible. In this subgroup, both partners affirmed that they had had no other partners since marriage, or at least not in the past few years. Most of the women in this age group said that they had married in early adolescence and had never had another partner. The final one-third of women said that dialogue had succeeded and their husbands agreed in principle to use condoms. What this meant in actual practice we were unable to discover. Methods of obtaining anonymous self-reports will have to be devised, taking into account the extremely limited literacy of poor and working class women. Couples in both the second and third groups agreed that their older children needed to be informed and some requested condoms for them.

The churchwomen requested that workshops be organized for husbands, adolescents, and young adult members of their households. While several mothers said that they could talk to their sexually active older children about AIDS and actually began to supply them with condoms, most felt constrained by traditional taboos against sharing intimate knowledge between parents and children. This does not mean that there is a blanket taboo across generations. Aunts, uncles, and grandparents are considered appropriate instructors by many. These relatives, however, may not be present or possess the necessary information. This was the case in elite homes as well, where parents requested that CONNAIS-SIDA hold workshops for their children and other young people living with them. Family-centered approaches offer ways to reach sexually active adolescents who are neither in school nor regularly employed.

Sex workers pointed to the need for accessible and affordable treatment for sexually transmitted diseases. And several women in the church group requested money for fees and transportation in order to obtain effective care for relief of persistent abdominal pain, which was unavailable in their neighborhood.[7] Because other sexually transmitted diseases, particularly those which cause genital ulcers, have been identified as a significant cofactor in HIV transmission, their treatment is essential to successful AIDS prevention. Not only are new services needed, but they must be free services, accessible to poor women in peripheral as well as central neighborhoods. Because treatment for sexually transmitted diseases is laden with cultural meaning and misperceptions, health workers will need assistance to provide sensitive, effective care.

The most pressing need identified by both women's groups is for income-generating activities so that women who cannot depend upon men to support them and their children can survive without providing sexual services to multiple partners. Both sex workers and churchwomen reported trying numerous other ways to enlarge family resources. Most have had scant success. Both groups drew up lists of needs and possibilities without arriving at a realistic plan of cooperative action that might be sustainable in the medium or long term, even with initial support from a funding agency.

One month following their evaluation, the church Mothers Club organized a festive meal for participants and trainers. Closing the proceedings, the minister advised the assembly that because AIDS is a divine retribution for sins, the righteous need not fear infection. A similar message was broadcast by the Protestant Bishop some days earlier. Future evaluation will show which of the competing messages, the moralistic one with its avoidance of realistic risk assessment or those developed by the group in collaboration with CONNAISSIDA, prevails.

Conclusion

Like so many other diseases produced by socioeconomic and political conditions, AIDS is a disease of development and underdevelopment. The virus is a biological event, the effects of which are magnified by the conditions of urbanization in African societies, distorted development, and the current world economic crisis. Linking macrolevel political economy to microlevel sociocultural analysis shows how women's survival strategies have turned into death strategies.

The two community groups with which we worked—the first an informal network, the second a local voluntary association—were invaluable in helping us to understand the social context and changing response to AIDS. The CONNAISSIDA experiment indicates that women perceive a need for AIDS information presented in an interactive setting. It also shows that by themselves, women cannot effect widespread AIDS prevention.

Breaking the chain of transmission will require rapid and widespread behavioral change. Yet directed social change is one of the most complex and least understood aspects of sociocultural dynamics. Several public health advisors take the view (in manuscripts with restricted distribution) that cost savings can be achieved by targeting AIDS prevention information to professional sex workers who comprise the highest risk group. While this would protect future clients, the fact that between 10 and 30 percent of all sexually active men and women are already HIV positive in some cities of Central and East Africa rules out attempts to find cheap solutions. Moreover, if sex workers are to use condoms regularly, their partners must accept them. The problem of relative social power and powerlessness has been neglected by these advisers who appear to be seeking a quick technological fix.

AIDS prevention is both personal and political. Change to safer sexual practices involves much more than the adoption of an unpopular imported technology; it involves redefinition of gendered social roles and change in the socioeconomic conditions that have contributed to the rapid spread of AIDS in the region.

Action-research and interviews found many women psychologically prepared to accept behavioral changes which would limit the risks of infection for themselves and their children. Yet their subordinate status in relation to their partners made it dangerous for some to attempt to negotiate sex. Without widespread implementation of community-based prevention strategies, we can expect differences in the incidence of new HIV infections to follow existing differences in socioeconomic power and access to information. We have shown that among marginal and powerless groups, increased knowledge and some behavior change can be triggered by education based on an active, participatory learning method. Sustained change requires consistent support from other levels of the society, however. It requires change among men, particularly those of high status. Culturally appropriate empowering education is one necessary but not sufficient part of AIDS prevention or of any health and development strategy. The limited long-term success of CONNAISSIDA's experiment with sex workers and churchwomen is a reminder that communication systems are social systems and exhibit the same hierarchically structured patterns as the wider society.

Married or "free," women of all classes are at risk for AIDS. We have seen that women's efforts at risk reduction are stymied by the refusal of many men to abandon the sexual prerogatives that the social structure provides. These prerogatives are integral to the society that developed out of the colonial encounter, with its characteristic political economy and patriarchal culture. With few opportunities for economic independence, most women are vulnerable to sexual demands by men with superior social power.

The rapid spread of AIDS in the region results from the gendered structure of inequality within a stagnant economy in which accumulation by international capital and a local ruling class leaves the majority pauperized. Within the poor majority, as within the privileged and middle classes, most women are economically and politically subordinated, their autonomy restricted, and their choices circumscribed. While some men are able to make changes, many have not yet recognized the need to do so, which means that AIDS will continue to spread and women will be blamed for spreading infection.

The socioeconomic constraints to behavioral change cannot be ignored, for they continue to limit the possibilities of even highly motivated individuals to alter their behavior. In the final analysis, effective AIDS control in Africa will require changing the economic and social status of women. Women's economic independence, their personal autonomy, and their control over interpersonal relations, including their power to negotiate sex, must be increased in order to stop AIDS.

· 12 ·

Taking Women Seriously

Toward Democratic Health Care in Africa

MEREDETH TURSHEN

HALF THE WORLD'S population is female, and three-quarters of the third world's population is composed of women and children who are still everywhere cared for by women. Women and children are the main users of health services, and women are the main providers of health care—within their families, in biomedical facilities (as nursing and support personnel), and often in traditional health care systems as well (mostly as tradition- al birth attendants) (Pizurki, Mejia, Butter, and Ewart 1987). It is logical to suggest, on the basis of these facts, that there can be no democratic health care in Africa until governments take women seriously. Government recognition of women is not a sufficient condition of democratic health care, but it is a necessary one. The task here is to define democratic health care and to describe what taking women seriously entails. The points are set out in the framework of a typology of African governments and illustrated by examples from the West African experience, particularly from Burkina Faso, Gabon, Mali, Mauritania, Niger, Senegal, and Western Sahara.

Health care is one of the first social services offered by every independent government, whether to prove that it can carry on the services provided by the former regime or to distinguish itself by democratizing the health system. Race and class are often burning issues in the early days of independence: the access of blacks to segregated medical care and the access of the poor to a system catering to the privileged are items high on the agenda of the new ministry of health. Gender is rarely addressed as such; the men who run the government and the medical men who run the health system assume that women will be covered by services that reach the blacks and the poor.

Most colonial governments provided some type of maternal and child health services. As Ladjali remarks in Chapter Eight, the French colonists saw maternal and child health as a Christian act of charity (even in Muslim countries). Competing European churches of different denominations often ran these services, sometimes with government support; in Tanzania, for example, the British colonial government subsidized the medical missions (Turshen 1984). The churches shared an interest in religious conversion and a concern for child health, which outweighed their investment in women's health. As Ladjali notes in the case of Algeria, many governments continued to offer these services after independence, initially with no change in orientation.

In those countries in which a black elite replaces the white regime, the health needs of the majority of the population are not likely to be much better served than they were before independence. Despite widely varied ways of conjugating new and traditional power structures, governments of this type retained the colonial health system, which was an urban service, based in hospitals, providing curative care, reliant upon sophisticated technology, and devoted to the chronic conditions of the privileged, only now the privileged were black. In Gabon, for example, twenty years after independence, 78 percent of the health budget was still allocated to hospitals in the three main cities (Port-Gentil, Libreville, and Franceville), and 62 percent of the physicians and one-fourth of the hospitals and medical centers were located in Libreville, the capital city, in which only 22 percent of the population lived (République Française 1981, 31-32). Most deaths in Libreville were thought to be due to cardiovascular disease (République Gabonaise 1980, 22).

Medical technology develops with a logic of its own, independent of the population's needs; it serves the government and its influential medical corps as an instrument of power. Witness, for example, the construction of an expensive International Center for Medical Research in Franceville, created to study the problems of infertility in Gabon. While sexually transmitted diseases go untreated and the infant mortality rate hovers above one hundred per thousand live births, the government is reinforcing its popularity by catering to urban elites concerned with low birth rates. Instead of extending primary health care to the rural areas, the government will probably fund experiments in *in vitro* fertilization ("test-tube babies").

Under governments of this type, the majority of rural poor, whose health needs include food, water, a clean environment, protection from the prevalent communicable diseases, occupational health care, and basic gynecological, obstetric, and pediatric services, are excluded from the redistribution of inherited colonial goods and services. Because women are overrepresented among the rural poor, they suffer disproportionately from the failure to redistribute equitably the new nation's inheritance.

Those countries in which a socialist government replaces the capitalist regime at the very least will pay lip service to the ideals of equitable redistribution. Mali, for instance, opted for a socialist path at independence in 1960. Periodically, as in 1976 after the UNICEF/World Health Organization conference on primary health care, the government affirms its intention to distribute health services equitably (OMS 1980, 459). In reality there is an extreme geographical imbalance: more than half of all doctors and almost two-thirds of midwives are located in Bamako, the capital city, in which there is one hospital bed for every 433 inhabitants; nationally there is one bed for every 1,634 inhabitants (UNICEF 1989, 186, 230). In 1983, the health system served an estimated 15 percent of Mali's 7.6 million people, 80 percent of whom live in rural areas; fifteen is also the meager percentage of women assisted in childbirth by a trained attendant (WHO 1989, 11). Urban women are better served than their rural sisters: in Mali, 69 percent of urban women receive prenatal care as against 14 percent of rural women, and 74 percent of urban women are assisted in childbirth by a trained attendant as against 12 percent of rural women (WHO 1989, 11). Condé (1983, 113) says of the *matrones*, the traditional Malian midwives, that their medical training is practically nil. The result is very high rates of maternal mortality. UNICEF (1989, 179) estimates that half of all deaths of women fifteen to forty-five years old are related to pregnancy and childbirth.

The basic elements of a democratic health service include—as a minimum—equitable distribution of food, water, sanitation, preventive health services, and free curative medical care to women, children, and men of all social classes in rural and urban areas. But democratic health care entails a process as well as a provision of services. Some regimes, such as that in Tanzania after the Arusha Declaration of 1967, which pledged the country to African socialism, tried to pay attention to issues of democratic process, for example by reversing the usual top-down planning process (Turshen 1984).

When wars of liberation are waged, the democratization of health services often begins before independence in areas reclaimed from the colonial power. It is a matter of necessity to care for wounded fighters and of strategic importance to extend health services to the people. Services designed for military campaigns are traditionally curative rather than preventive, and hospital-rather than community-oriented.[1] Socialist liberation movements, whether in Cuba, Vietnam, or Eritrea, have generally placed heavy emphasis on community health care (Sabo and Kibirige 1989). Where women's liberation is part of the commitment of the socialist movement, preventive services for mothers and children are organized as an extension of community health care. Eritrea appears to have done more than any previous liberation movement by using both maternal and child health care and training in the provision of health services to empower women. In the refugee camps of Western Sahara, nurses aides, who receive a year of on-the-job training in the national hospital, circulate among the tents. Each encampment has a person in charge of health who selects one health worker for each row of tents. Visits are systematic and reinforce camp hygiene. The aides advise pregnant women to seek prenatal care, carefully explaining its importance, and encourage them to give birth in hospital (Perregaux 1990, 53-54).

The war experience does not necessarily dictate the design of the service that is offered after the war is won. The new government encounters formidable obstacles to the delivery of rural health services, which are related to the colonial legacy of urban predominance in planning: in general, disparities between urban and rural areas have tended to increase since independence, as part of the wider trend to greater class differentiation (Turshen 1984). The new government must overcome an infrastructure oriented to the metropolitan center. To guarantee food and water, lines of communication that run from mines and plantations to the ports must be reconfigured to serve the regional distribution of goods and services; land concentrations must be broken up and reformed; the commercial production of export crops must be supplanted by food crops for domestic consumption; credit must be extended creatively to rural households, including those headed by women; new technologies must be made available to all farmers, male and female; and water diverted to mines and plantations must be shared with subsistence households.

A whole new tier of primary health care facilities must be built to serve rural communities, and it must be integrated into the secondary and tertiary care system. In some countries, for example Gabon, the principle of free health services is compromised by the demand that primary health care be self-sufficient; in other words, peasants must pay for the construction and maintenance of clinics and for supplies and equipment, whereas urban health services remain free of charge. This type of primary health care program makes peasants pay for the physical consequences of their exploitation and enables urban elites to avoid sharing the benefits of advanced medical technology. The existence of a government health service is not the equivalent socialized health care, even if the private practice of medicine (including some traditional medicine), which drains the government service of resources, has somehow been eliminated. Socialist health care implies the democratic participation of users of the system and of all workers in the planning and operation of the system, through representative structures such as trade unions.

The staffing of rural health services and their integration into a socialized and nationalized system will not take place without a reform of education. The educational system must not only be expanded but also redirected to serve democratic needs and aspirations. The difficulties of redesigning elitist school systems that produce professionals and office workers for urban employment cannot be underestimated (Turshen 1984). Current social rewards reinforce the old educational structure, and the incumbent generation of vested professionals and educators resists change. Medical education, perverted for decades to produce clinical specialists, must be revised to train generalists, who are familiar with rural health problems and prepared to work in teams of public health professionals under conditions of scarcity, not necessarily as team leaders. The individualistic, entrepreneurial orientation must be replaced by a social orientation informed by economic realities, and health professionals must be equipped to cope realistically, within the context of a representative political structure.

And even this recipe is out of date. Who is preparing to deal with the health effects of new forms of social stress, environmental degradation, and labor exploitation?

Reproductive Health

The first problem of defining democratic health care is deciding who will control the definition of health. Maoists proclaim that professionals must be "red and expert," meaning that political imperatives take precedence over technical requirements and are used to reinterpret them. This formula begs the question because it leaves the definition of health in the hands of those who proffer health services and does not put control of the definition into the hands of those who use the services.

Although gender is rarely on the agenda in the early days of designing a new health service for the independent nation, governments do take an interest in their female population in specific circumstances: for example, when more workers enter the labor force than the job market can absorb; when the number of unemployed reaches dangerous levels and threatens the stability of the government; when the number of children and elderly that must be supported by working adults becomes an intolerable burden; and when the demand for food, housing, education, and social services outstrips the ability, or will, of the government to provide them. Then, suddenly, governments take an interest in women, or rather in that narrow aspect of women's lives that concerns reproduction. For example, in a 1986 address the president of Niger compared his country's rapid population growth with its slow rate of economic growth and said, *"Excusez-moi, mes soeurs, mais vous pondez trop!"* ("Excuse me, sisters, but you give birth too often!" Quoted in Monimart 1989, 196.) Niger's 1987-1991 development plan places the need to control population growth at the head of the list of major challenges facing the country. It is interesting to recall that population density in Niger is 5.3 inhabitants per square kilometer, whereas it is 102 in France and 359 in Holland.

Population control is a predictable, simplistic response to complex problems of economic development, as Lindsay shows for mineral-rich Namibia in Chapter Nine and as Ladjali shows for oil-dependent Algeria. Governments draw a double advantage from this approach—they please international organizations and bilateral donors by adopting antinatalist policies, and they maintain control over the female population by reducing women to their reproductive functions.

Population programs are variously disguised. They are promoted as maternal and child health care (see the recommendations of the World Health Organization [OMS 1971]); as *espacement des naissances* (see Ladjali on Algeria, and Monimart [1989, 187-190] on Burkina Faso) and as family planning. Tunisia is a good example of the latter (see Ennaïfer 1988). Abortion on demand is another disguise. The Japanese government used abortion after World War II to bring the birth rate down from 33 per 1,000 population in 1949 to 17 per 1,000 in 1957. In 1955 a record 1,170,000 abortions were performed under Japan's Eugenic Protection Law; and in 1970 the government reported that 42 percent of married women had undergone an abortion in Japan

(Wagatsuma 1971, 30-31). Some governments use sterilization to control population growth: at the height of its campaign in 1976, the Indian health services performed eight million sterilizations (Landman 1977, 102). Other governments resort to hysterectomies; Ward (1986) describes how doctors in Catholic parishes of Louisiana performed hysterectomies on African-American women who wanted birth contol. The most recent addition to this list is AIDS protection: in response to a report of fifteen hundred cases of AIDS in Côte d'Ivoire, the U.S. government sent three million condoms and promised five million more (*Le Monde* 10 January 1990). In Chapter Eleven, Schoepf et al. report promoting condoms for this purpose in Zaire.

In Burkina Faso, the official policy is ostensibly one of pregnancy spacing in order to preserve the health of mother and child, but the objectives of the national family planning plan include education in the interaction between population and development and the benefits of contraception as a means of combatting, among other ills, delinquency and unemployment (Monimart 1989, 187). It is interesting to observe that only governments with pronatalist policies undertake programs to lighten the burdens of child rearing. Barbara Brown (1987) describes the elaborate social benefits that South Africa pays to white mothers in order to encourage them to bear more children.

The medicalization of reproduction, which is after all a normal and not a pathological life process, is a striking aspect of the government response to economic woes. The same objective could be achieved in other ways. Social controls such as later age at marriage for women are an equally effective—and, in several parts of Africa, traditional—means of lowering the birth rate (Turshen 1984). Few countries enforce a legal age of marriage even when they have fixed a minimum age; in Senegal, for instance, the minimum age is sixteen years, but the law is frequently broken (Monimart 1989, 199). The age of first marriage may actually be dropping in societies in which girls wed soon after puberty, because the worldwide trend is toward earlier menarche. On the other hand, it is encouraging to note, as Ladjali does, that education tends to raise the marriage age for women and men.

Equally striking, and completely paradoxical, is the limited interest governments and their international advisors take in women's health: even maternal and child health services are concerned narrowly with pregnancy outcomes, that is to say with the health of the woman only as the child bearer. For example, of ten risks associated with human reproduction cited by UNICEF, the World Health Organization, and the World Bank (1987, 35), only one—maternal mortality—actually affects the woman. All of the others affect children—diseases transmitted sexually to the fetus (syphilis, hepatitis B, AIDS); abortion (as a cause of fetal death); malnourished newborns; lack of neonatal care for newborns; stillbirths (in women over forty); unattended home births (as a cause of perinatal death); neonatal death; malnourished infants; and a subsequent pregnancy within one year, which increases the first child's mortality risk by 75 percent.

If the function of childbearing is biological, the role of child rearer, of being a mother, is a specifically social status, and in many places it is the only institutionalized social status for women. In Niger, for example, a high official opened the second congress of Nigerien women in 1979 with these words: *"Vous êtes femmes, faites pour l'intérieur .... Nous sommes hommes, faits pour l'extérieur."* ("You women belong in the home .... Men are made for the public sphere." Quoted in Monimart 1989, 217).

The logic of defining women by their reproductive function is circular, in the sense that women caught up in this circuit are often deprived of the economic autonomy needed to leave it. Recognition of women's productive contributions might confer this independence. In Niger, the female share of nonagricultural employment was 7 percent in 1986 (Standing 1989, 1083). In Algeria, it is 4 percent. Guillaume shows in Chapter Ten that these low figures rarely reflect the reality of women's many jobs, and that the specific techniques of multiple-round surveys are needed to elicit accurate information.

Women who are not paid for their work have limited decision-making powers, within the family and within society, including the power to control their own fertility. Ladjali describes the complex negotiations involving husbands, mothers-in-law, and brothers-in-law that take place when Algerian women decide to limit the size of their families. Vock (1988) suggests that women may resort to subterfuge (for example, use contraception secretly) to avoid pregnancy. A recent study of women attending family planning clinics near Paris found that West African women could rarely obtain their husbands' consent to contraceptive practice (Turshen et al., forthcoming).

The more children a woman has, the less likely she is to enter paid employment or become an active participant in the political institutions that govern her country, as Loewenson observes in Zimbabwe. Guillaume describes the complicated arrangements Ivorian women make to entrust their children to other women in order to balance their productive and reproductive tasks. In addition to issues of government policy, all of the arrangements women make to balance their productive and reproductive obligations raise questions about sexual politics in the household, which are discussed in the chapter on gender and health.

Women who live in urban areas have a life experience different from that of their rural sisters. The gulf between the two can be quite large, which has implications for, among others, the relevance of women's associations founded by urban women and serving women in the countryside. During a meeting of the National Revolutionary Council on women's liberation, a peasant woman in Burkina Faso addressed Josephine Ouédraogo, Minister for Family Affairs in Thomas Sankara's government, in these terms:

> I dare to speak in order to tell you that everything you say about women's sufferings is true and your sincerity is touching. However, you, our city sisters, you can never understand our lives in the bush. The problem [polygamy] that you raise, it is just the smoke seen from a distance, because you cannot see the fire that causes the smoke. . . . Peasant women that we are, we will never fight against our husbands and co-wives: they are too useful to us! (quoted in Kanse 1989, 71)

Urban women who are recent migrants from the countryside face special difficulties of adaptation if they lose the status of productive worker, which conferred some economic independence and freedom of movement. Cities offer limited wage-earning possibilities, especially to women with little or no formal education. The alternatives are petty commodity production and the informal sector (Bujra 1988). On the other hand, some women experience the move to the city as liberating because they are freed of the constraints imposed by traditional society. "For me, for my maternal grandmother, the city is liberating: social pressures are not as strong and there are fewer taboos of all sorts." (Interview with a Togolese university instructor quoted in Deniel 1985, 101) Certainly, girls reared in town will have greater educational opportunities than girls who grow up on farms, and education tends to modify aspirations, enabling girls to break with traditional models of womanhood and to envisage other identities.

Among the social pressures that trap women in subordinate roles, religious traditions are often predominant and are frequently manipulated by governments to their advantage. Religious ideologies exercise social control of women through their definitions of sexuality. A return to fundamentalism is evident in all the major world religions and it affects women in both developed and underdeveloped countries. North and south of the Sahara, women experience in different ways the rise of Islamic fundamentalism. Keita (1983, 102-103) claims that Nigerien women are crushed by the weight of Islam, and that they alone bear the inconveniences of fundamentalist religious practices. Fatimatou Allali, the first woman to be elected to the political bureau of Polisario and former secretary-general of the National Union of Sahrawi Women, sees colonialism, rather than Islam, at the root of women's oppression; colonization and urban settlement forced Sahrawi women into a dependent situation in homes that became veritable prisons for a formerly free and nomadic population. Allali sees Islam as a unifying force in the refugee community (Perregaux 1990, 73).

Among unemployed urban youth, Islamic fundamentalism may be a response to the failure of development strategies. Amin (1989, 15) estimates that half of the potentially active men in African towns have no fixed income and constitute an unabsorbable reserve of unemployed and semiemployed workers. In this context it is not surprising that Islamic fundamentalists militate against coeducation, or that young men perceive the education of girls as leading to increased competition for scarce jobs. In the current economic climate, in which the total number of jobs is falling, men resent rising levels of female employment. According to Standing (1989, 1080), growth in the use of female labor around the world is absolute and relative, and many jobs traditionally dominated by men are being "feminized." Religious fundamentalists oppose the adoption of family codes that favor women and press governments to repeal those reforms previously adopted; in Islamic states such as Algeria, they demand the substitution of the Sharia, which is Islamic law. Behind these pressures is the challenging new phenomenon of literate young women claiming a place in economies that are often shrinking rather than growing. Fundamentalism is a backlash and, in this sense, it represents a measure of women's success, rather than an indication of women's failure. But of course women lose out under these intolerant, rigid, and antidemocratic regimes.

Taking Women Seriously

A woman-centered definition of reproductive health begins with a redefinition of woman's place in society, which requires a reexamination of women's access to paid employment, political participation, and education. Additionally, in rural areas, it involves changes in household decision-making patterns, described by Mebrahtu in Chapter Six as pivotal in the lives of Yoruba-speaking women in Nigeria, as well as changes in women's access to labor (Roberts 1988). It also entails calling into question dominant ideologies such as religion, and the codification of conservative traditions in legislation and in family policy.

The revolution of August 1983 in Burkina Faso, which brought Thomas Sankara to power, entailed a reexamination of women's roles and responsibilities. Until that date, according to Alimata Salembéré, secretary of state for culture in the Ministry of Environment and Tourism in 1988 (quoted in Tarrab 1989, 43), women were not allowed to speak in public assemblies—even in the rural areas from which men migrate and leave their wives in charge of their households. After 1983, women assumed ministerial posts—

and not just those such as women's affairs traditionally reserved for token appointments (ibid.). In 1987 the minister of the budget was a woman; in 1988 the minister for environment and tourism, the secretary of state for social action, and the secretary of state for culture were all women (ibid., 68). Many women occupied management level posts in the administrations of Thomas Sankara and the current president, Blaise Compaoré, in the provinces as well as in Ouagadougou, the capital. Women serve in the army; one year of military service in SERNAPO (*Service national populaire*) is obligatory between the ages of twenty and thirty-five years and is a prerequisite for public employment (ibid., 73). The 1983 revolution also brought a repeal of customary law (for a detailed review see Turshen 1989, 100-102). Revolutionary tribunals, composed of professional judges and competent citizens, which include women, have replaced the customary courts (Tarrab 1989, 73-74).

If women are to serve and be served equally with men in a democratic health service, sexist colonial legislation must be repealed. These laws control women's age of majority, access to and conditions of paid employment, freedom of movement, access to education and technical training, access to abortion, and access to contraceptive information and devices. In Senegal, women who want paid work must obtain their husband's consent, even though women workers are not a new phenomenon and women have always been active in Senegalese economic life (Savané 1983, 114). The Government of Mali repealed some of the 1920 French colonial laws, which banned all birth control; but only therapeutic abortions are legal in Mali, and access to modern contraceptive methods requires one's husband's permission (Monimart 1989, 193). In Niger, too, only married women have access to contraception and only with their husband's consent (Keita 1983, 108).

Cumulatively, legislation such as family codes defines women and institutionalizes their social status. Women and their bona fide representatives must rewrite marriage laws and family codes, dealing simultaneously with bodies of colonial and customary law. Of course one cannot stop at the adoption of legislation; the laws must be applied. In Mali, for example, the newly independent government, under the pressure of women's organizations led by

Awa Keita, an anticolonial militant (Condé 1983, 112), adopted an innovative marriage law in 1962. The new law improved women's status by requiring women's consent in marriage, by assuring the legality of civil weddings, and by affirming women's right to sue for divorce, to have custody of their children, and to receive alimony. For twenty-five years, however, Malian women have been waiting for the law to be applied (Monimart 1989, 215).

To repeal outdated laws that no longer correspond to social realities is a first step, but most countries need to reach beyond conventional solutions. One example of creative thinking is Thomas Sankara's attempt to install a family wage, which would entitle women in Burkina Faso to a portion of the salary earned by their husbands.[2] Women were to receive their part of the wage in the form of coupons, which they could exchange in state stores for rice, sugar, soap, and other necessities (Tarrab 1989, 75). Sankara justified this measure with the claim that "some men transform their wives into housekeepers without paying them the wages of a domestic" (Kanse 1989, 70). As an interim measure, in a country in which 97.6 percent of women are illiterate, the family wage might have improved the lot of some women (of course there is always the danger that such payments will keep women in a limited, stereotypical role). Whatever the failures of implementation (most subsistence peasant households had no waged worker and were not eligible), the conception is in advance of most social legislation in Africa.

In some countries, there is an issue of separation of church and state: one is hard pressed to name a theocracy in which women are not subordinate; theocracy and democracy are by definition mutually exclusive categories. Mauritania is one of several African Islamic states that apply the Sharia, the body of Moslem law, which segregates women from men and assigns a minor's status to women.

Women's organizations are clearly central to this reform project, not only women's cooperative efforts in executing the day-to-day strategies upon which the continent's survival depends, but also formal organizations. According to Chazan (1989, 190), marginalization is the dominant image of such groups in Africa. Many political parties, including socialist parties, have women's auxiliaries (one example is the Senegalese socialist party); but few of them are autonomous or genuinely grassroots organizations. The grassroots groups tend to be small, loosely structured, and detached from the power aparatus (ibid.). Alongside the proliferation of women's groups is the development of large umbrella organizations which tend to be fragile. One such umbrella is the Federation of Senegalese Women's Associations (FAFS), which comprises two hundred independent organizations. The creation of radical groups that have a more focused political agenda is a response to the fragility of large umbrella organizations; in Senegal, for example, feminists founded a controversial liberation group, Yewwu-Yewwi PLF,[3] in 1984 in reaction to FAFS (Monimart 1989, 218). Chazan (1989, 191) suggests that women's collective action is at the frontiers of formal political arrangements, raising the conceptual possibility that women occupy the interstices of political power in many African states; "by filling in political spaces, they may constitute an important bridge between official institutions and informal political processses and economic activities."

The failure of governments—of whatever political stripe—to give women a legitimate voice has not stopped political struggles, as several chapters in this volume show, notably those on South Africa by Lubanga and Khan. South Africa is perhaps an extreme case of provocation. In a study of women's participation in workers' struggles, Nomvete (1984) discusses the unionization of South African domestic workers in the early 1980s. In the Western Cape, women formed the Domestic Workers Association; in the Eastern Cape, they organized the Domestic Workers and Salesladies Association; and in Natal, they created the National Union of Domestic Workers. In December 1981, these organizations met and drew up a common charter, which included demands for minimum wage rates, an eight-hour day, paid leave, decent living conditions for live-in workers, and the specific charge that "no domestic servant shall be dismissed as a result of pregnancy or illness" (ibid., 112). Nomvete thinks that the trend to employ servants on a daily basis has placed women who commute to work in close contact with one another, which has enabled them to organize.

In conclusion, to speak seriously of democratic health care in Africa implies taking women seriously, not as targets of population control programs, which reduce women to the single dimension of their reproductive organs, but as productive members of society with equal political rights, social status, and economic value.

Notes

Notes to Chapter One

1. Technically, total fertility is the number of children each woman would bear if she lived to the end of her childbearing years and bore children at each age in accordance with prevailing age-specific fertility rates.

Notes to Chapter Three

1. Rural councils are the local government administrative units that cover the large-scale farming areas. They exist together with the urban councils and with the district councils that cover the peasant areas.
2. The General Agricultural and Plantation Workers Union (GAPWUZ) coexisted with a splinter union, Zimbabwe Agricultural Workers Union (ZAWU), in the early 1980s, until GAPWUZ was officially registered and ZAWU ceased to exist.

Notes to Chapter Four

1. Wayfarers are the South African equivalent of Girl Scouts and Girl Guides. Instead of unionizing, African women were advised by SATNA officials to form a troop of Girl Scouts!

Notes to Chapter Five

1. I would like to express my gratitude to my husband, for his continued support and encouragement in the writing of this chapter, and to Dr. Zubie Hamed for useful discussions on the dermatological problems.
2. Athol Fugard's moving play, *Master Harald and the Boys,* captures exactly this situation but with male characters (Editor's note).

Notes to Chapter Seven

1. The six countries are Cameroon, Ghana, Kenya, Lesotho, Senegal, and Sudan.
2. Female circumcision is not an Islamic custom. It is widely practiced in twenty-four countries of sub-Saharan Africa, and there are reports of some cases in seven others. Infibulation, the most extensive operation, is widely practiced in five countries and in parts of four others, including Christianized Ethiopia and Eritrea (Paquot 1983, 341). In North Africa, circumcision is limited to Egypt. It is unknown in many parts of the Middle East, but practiced in Iraq, Jordan, Saudi Arabia, Yemen, and some parts of Syria (Minces 1990, 97).

Notes to Chapter Nine

1. According to the World Health Organization, drugs used in the treatment of tuberculosis (such as Rifampicin) lower the blood level of the progestin contained in injectable contraceptives such as Depo-Provera and inhibit their contraceptive effect (Susan Holck and David Back, personal communications with the Editor, June 1990). The physicians in Namibia may not have been aware of this recent finding, which is not as well known as the interaction between anti-TB drugs and the estrogen component of oral contraceptives. (Editor's note)

Notes to Chapter Eleven

1. Earlier versions of this chapter were presented at the First International Conference on AIDS Education and Information, Ixtapa, Mexico, October 16, 1988; at the Conference on Women, Development and Health, Michigan State University, October 23, 1988; and submitted to *Social Science and Medicine* January 15, 1989. Grateful acknowledgment is made to the Government of Zaire's Conseil Executif, the Rockefeller Foundation, the Wenner Gren Foundation for Anthropological Research, and OXFAM (U.K.) for their generous support, as well as to research assistants Eke Tukumbe, Latchung Amen, Ngirabakunzi N'mukulira, and Pika Nianga. None of these institutions or individuals is in any way responsible for the data or interpretations in this chapter.

2. References to the biomedical literature are omitted to save space. They can be found in Schoepf and Schoepf (1981) and in Koch-Weser and Vanderschmidt (1988).

3. This survey is an example of the limitations of questionnaire methods in eliciting data on sensitive subjects.

4. Locally these sex workers are called *mingando*, a disparaging term that refers to their ethnic origin, poverty, and virtually exclusive reliance on sex with multiple partners for a livelihood. They reported receiving the equivalent of 50 to 60 U.S. cents per encounter. Similarly poor sex workers live scattered throughout the city.

5. Used in a mixed group of community development workers, this role play missed the mark when male participants failed to perceive that the woman portrayed was a chief, despite her ways of sitting, moving, and speaking which normally convey power and authority in Central Africa. However, their blindness opened the door to a new exercise around which to structure learning about gender roles.

6. As advised by the senior author (June 1986 and subsequently), the project promotes condoms as protection from AIDS, rather than as a contraceptive. According to the project's Marketing Director, a former CONNAISSIDA assistant, sales in Kinshasa reached 300,000 after one year of operation (Mivumbi 1988).

7. A new clinic treating women for sexually transmitted diseases was opened by the biomedical AIDS research group, Projet SIDA, in a popular entertainment district in 1988. Forty percent of the first five hundred patients were found to be HIV positive by mid- year (Dr. Nzila, personal communication, July 1988).

Notes to Chapter Twelve

1. Losses due to preventable diarrhea and malaria were usually much higher than those due to battle wounds.
2. The negative side of the family wage can be observed in Algeria: the newly elected Front Islamique du Salut decreed a family wage to keep women at home and out of the workforce. My fear is that it will eventually be used to justify the curtailment of education for girls.
3. These words mean "prendre conscience et rompre" or, in the classical formulation, rise up and break the chains that bind ye.

References

Acharya, M., and L. Bennet. 1983. "Women and Subsistence Sector: Economic Participation and Household Decision Making in Nepal." *World Bank Staff Working Paper* No. 526. Washington, D.C.: The World Bank.

Adeyokunnu, T. O. 1981. "Women and Agriculture in Nigeria." Addis Abeba: United Nations Economic Commission for Africa.

AIM. 1989a. (Agência de Informaçâo de Moçambique). Reproduced in Mozambique Information Office News Review No. 149/50, London.

AIM. 1989b. Reproduced in Mozambique Information Office News Review No. 153, London.

Allison, C. 1985. "Women, Land, Labour and Survival: Getting Some Basic Facts Straight." *IDS Bulletin* 16(3):24-30.

Amin, S. 1989. *La Faillite du Développement en Afrique et dans le Tiers-Monde: Une Analyse Politique.* Paris: L'Harmattan.

Andersson, Neil. 1984. *Health Sector Policy Options for Independent Namibia.* Lusaka: United Nations Institute for Namibia.

Ay, P., and F. Nweke. 1984. "Women in Farm Production and Research." A Paper Presented at the Workshop on Women in Agriculture in West Africa. Organized by ILCA and IITA, May 7-9.

Barker, E. 1979. "Dimensions of Future Unemployment and Prospects for Wage Sector Employment in Zimbabwe." *Zimbabwe Journal of Economics* 1(1) March.

Beneria, L. 1982. "Accounting for Women's Work." In *Women and Development: The Sexual Division of Labor in Rural Societies*, 119-147. New York: Praeger Scientific.

Berio, A. J. 1984. "The Analysis of Time Allocation and Activity Patterns in Nutrition and Rural Development Planning." *Food and Nutrition Bulletin* 6(1):53-68.

Bertrand, J. T., M. Bakutuvwidi, L. M. Kinavwidi, and D. Balowa. 1989. "Knowledge of AIDS, Sexual Behavior and Condom Use in the Context of AIDS Prevention." Report to USAID. Washington, D.C., mimeo.

Bleiberg, F. M., T. A. Brun, and S. Goihman. 1980. "Duration of Activities and Energy Expenditure of Female Farmers in Dry and Rainy Seasons in Upper Volta." *British Journal of Nutrition* 43:71-82.

Borcherds, M. G. 1958. "The South African Nursing Act. An account of events leading up to and subsequent to the passing of the South African Nursing Act No. 69 of 1957." *International Nursing Review* July, 33.

Boserup, E. 1970. *Women's Role in Economic Development*. New York: St. Martin's Press.

Brown, Barbara. 1980. "Some Aspects of Women and Health." In *Women's Role in Development in Botswana*. Government of Botswana, Ministry of Agriculture, Rural Sociology Series.

———. 1987. "Facing the Black Peril: the Politics of Population Control in South Africa." *Journal of South African Studies* 13(2).

Brown, K. H. et al. 1988. "Consumption of Weaning Foods from Fermented Cereals in Kwara State, Nigeria." In *Improving Young Child Feeding in Eastern and Southern Africa: Household-Level Food Technology* edited by D. A. S. Moses and O. G. Schmidt. Ottawa, Canada: IDRC.

Brownmiller, Susan. 1975. *Against Our Will*. New York: Simon and Schuster.

Brun, T., F. Bleiberg, and S. Goihman. 1981. "Energy Expenditure of Male Farmers in Dry and Rainy Seasons in Upper Volta." *British Journal of Nutrition* 45:67-75.

Buvinic, M., J. Graeff, and J. Leslie. 1987. "Individual and Family Choices for Child Survival and Development: A Framework for Research in Sub-Saharan Africa." Washington, D.C.: ICRW.

Bwititi, T. and R. Loewenson. 1985. *Report of a Facility-based Survey of Pesticide Poisoning*. Harare: Mininstry of Health, mimeo.

Bwititi, T. et al. 1987. "Health Hazards of Organophosphate Use among Farmworkers in the Large Scale Farming Sector." *Central African Journal of Medicine* 33(5):120-126.

Caldwell, J., P. Caldwell, and P. Quiggin. 1989. "Disaster in an Alternative Civilization: The Social Dimensions of Aids in Sub- Saharan Africa." Canberra: National Centre for Epidemiology and Population Health.

Carp, C. 1983. "Seasonality, Women's Work, and Health." *Mothers and Children: Bulletin on Infant Feeding and Maternal Nutrition* 3(3):1-3.

Cashman, K. 1986. "The Yoruba Farmer and Her Household: Changing Agricultural Production in Yorubaland." An ILCA Report, Ibadan, Nigeria.

Central Statistical Office. 1985. *Main Demographic Features of the Population of Zimbabwe*. Harare: Government Printers.

———. 1986. *Statistical Yearbook 1985*. Harare: Government Printers.

———. 1988. *Statistical Yearbook 1987*. Harare: Government Printers.

Chambers, R. 1983. "Health, Agriculture, and Rural Poverty: Why Seasons Matter." *The Journal of Development Studies* 18(2):217-238.

Chambers, R. Longhurst, D. Bradely, and R. Feachmen. 1979. "Seasonal Dimensions to Rural Poverty: Analysis and Practical Applications." Institute of Development Studies *Discussion Paper* #142. Brighton: University of Sussex.

Chikanza, I., D. Paxton, R. Loewenson, and R. Laing. 1981. "The Health Status of Farmworker Communities in Zimbabwe." *Central African Journal of Medicine* 27(5):155-169.

Clarke, D. 1975. "A Note on the Agricultural and Plantation Workers Union in Rhodesia, 1964-1973." *South African Labour Bulletin* 1(9):53-65.

Cliff, Julie and Abdul Razak Noormahomed. 1988. "Health as a Target: South Africa's Destabilization of Mozambique." *Social Science and Medicine* (7) 27:717-722.

Cock, Jacklyn. 1989. *Maids and Madams: Domestic Workers under Apartheid*. London: The Women's Press.

Commercial Farmers Union. 1986. "The Green Paper: Mimeo on Problems and Solutions in Commercial Farming in Zimbabwe." Harare: Government of Zimbabwe, mimeo.

Condé, Maryse. 1983. "Mali: Plutôt se changer en oiseaux?" In *Terre des Femmes* sous la direction d'Elisabeth Paquot, 112-114. Paris: La Découverte.

Cornia, Giovanni A., Richard Jolly, and Frances Stewart. 1987a. *Adjustment with a Human Face. Protecting the Vulnerable and Promoting Growth*. Oxford: Oxford University Press.

Cowles, Ruth. 1933. "The Bantu Nurses' Association." *South African Nursing Record* 20:233.

Critical Health. 1988. "A Historical Overview of Nursing Struggles in South Africa." October, 24:53-62.

———. 1988. "The Origins of Contemporary Nursing Organisation in South Africa." October, 24:4-12.

Cross, E. G. 1976. "Man, Management in Agriculture: Labour Costs and Productivity in Agriculture." *Rhodesian Journal of Economics* 10(4):184-187.

Deniel, Raymond. 1985. *Femmes des Villes Africaines.* Abidjan, Côte d'Ivoire: INADES Edition.

Diehl, L. 1982. "Smallholder Farming Systems with Yam in the Southern Guinea Savanna of Nigeria." German Agency for Technical Cooperation (GTZ), Eschborn, Germany.

Diop, R. 1988. "Le travail des enfants dans le secteur informel: une étude de quelques des centres de pourvoyeurs 'd'enfants loués' de la région de Bondoukou." Abidjan: Faculté de lettres et arts et sciences humaines, Département de sociologie. Mémoire de Diplôme d'Etudes Appliquées.

Direction de la Statistique. 1982. *Enquête démographique à passages répétés, 1978-1979, résultats définitifs.* Abidjan: Ministère du Plan et de l'Industrie.

———. 1984. *Enquête ivoirienne sur la fécondité, 1980-1981.* Rapport principal, volume 1, Analyse des principaux résultats. Abidjan: Ministère de l'Economie et des Finances.

Dumont, René. 1990. "L'Afrique noire est-elle perdue?" *Le Monde Diplomatique*, mai, 23.

Duncan, B. 1973. "The Wages and Labour Supply Position in European Agriculture." *Rhodesian Journal of Economics* 7:1-13.

Du Toit, F. P. 1977. "The Accommodation of Permanent Farm Labourers." *Rhodesian Agricultural Journal* Technical Bulletin 17. Salisbury: Government Printer.

Edholm, F., O. Harris, and K. Young. 1977. "Conceptualizing Women." *Critique of Anthropology* 9/10:116-130.

Edmunds, Marianna. 1981. "Population Dynamics and Migrant Labor in South Africa." In *And the Poor Get Children* edited by Karen L. Michaelson, 154-179. London: Monthly Review Press.

Eide, W. B. and F. C. Steady. 1980. "Individual and Social Energy Flows: Bridging Nutritional and Anthropological Thinking About Women's Work in Rural Africa, Theoretical Considerations." In *Nutritional Anthropology: Contemporary Approaches to Diet and Culture* edited by N. W. Jerome, R. F. Kandel, and G. H. Pelto, 61-84. New York: Redgrave Publishing Co.

Elago, Nashilongo and Lindy Kazombaue. 1987. "The Exploited Women in Namibia: a Testimony." In *Namibia in Perspective* edited by G. Totemeyer, V. Kandetu, and W. Werner, 196-204. Windhoek: The Council of Churches in Namibia.

Elson, Diane. 1987. *The Impact of Structural Adjustment on Women: Concepts and Issues.* IFAA 1987 Conference on the Impact of IMF and World Bank Policies on the People of Africa, London.

ENAF. 1987. *Enquête nationale sur la fécondité.* Alger: Ministère du Travail et des Affaires Sociales.

Engle, P. 1981. "Maternal Care, Maternal Substitutes, and Children's Welfare in the Developed and Developing Countries." Background Paper for Policy Round Table on The Interface Between Poor Women's Nurturing Roles and Productive Responsibilities. Washington, D.C.: ICRW.

Enloe, C. 1983. *Does Khaki Become You?* London: Pandora Press.

Ennaïfer, Rachida. 1988. "Tunisia Takes Stock." *People: IPPF Review of Population and Development.* 15(3):11-12.

Etienne, Mona. 1979. "Maternité sociale, rapports d'adoption et pouvoir de femmes chez les Baoulé (Côte d'Ivoire)." *L'Homme,* XIX (3-4):63-107.

———. 1987. "Rapports de sexe et de classe et mobilité socio-économique chez les Baoulé (Côte d'Ivoire)." *Anthropologie et sociétés* II(1):71-93.

Fadipe, N. A. 1970. *The Sociology of the Yoruba.* Ibadan, Nigeria: Ibadan University Press.

Fainzang, S. et O. Journet. 1988. *La Femme de Mon Mari: Anthropologie du Mariage Polygamique en Afrique et en France.* Paris: L'Harmattan.

FAO. 1987. "Women in African Food Production and Food Security." In *Food Policy: Integrating Supply, Distribution, and Consumption,* edited by J. P. Gittinger, J. Leslie, and C. Hoistington, 133-140. Baltimore: The Johns Hopkins University Press.

———. 1983. "Time Allocation Survey: A Tool for Anthropologists, Economists, and Nutritionists." In *Expert Consultation on Women in Food Production.* Rome: FAO.

———. 1979. "Women in Food Production, Food Handling, and Nutrition With Special Emphasis on Africa." A Report of the Protein Advisory Group of the UN. Rome: FAO.

Fapohunda, E. R. 1988. "The Nonpooling Household: A Challenge to Theory." In *Home Divided: Women and Income in the Third World,* edited by D. Dwyser and J. Bruce. Stanford: Stanford University Press.

Fiege, H. 1985. "Planification régionale et développement socio- économique de la région du sud-ouest de la Côte-d'Ivoire." Université de Cologne.

230 · References

Francisco, Antonio, Ana Maria Ribeiro, Marina Pancas, and Belmiro Baptista. 1987. *Estudo do Sistema de Mercado e Horticolas e Frutas e Impacto da Liberalização dos Preços.* (Study of the Fruit and Vegetable Market and the Impact of Price Liberalization). Maputo.

Freire, P. 1978. *Pedagogy in Process.* New York: Seabury.

Gabriel, Daniel. 1988. *The Effects of South African Aggression on Economic Infrastructures.* European Conference Against South African Aggression in Mozambique and Angola, Bonn.

Gardner, H. and B. McCoppin. 1986. "Vocation, Career or Both? Politicisation of Australian Nurses, Victoria 1984-1986." *Australian Journal of Advanced Nursing* 4:24-35.

General Agricultural and Plantation Workers Union of Zimbabwe. 1988. *Report on the National Workshop on Health and Safety in Large Scale Farming Areas.* Harare: GAPWUZ.

Gersony, Robert. 1988. *Summary of Mozambican Refugee Accounts of Principally Conflict-Related Experience in Mozambique.* Washington, D.C.: Bureau for Refugee Programs, U.S. Department of State.

Gevins, A. 1987. "Tackling Tradition: African Women Speak Out Against Female Circumcision." In *Third World, Second Sex* compiled by Miranda Davies, 244-249. Vol. 2. London: Zed Books.

Goldschmidt-Clermont, L. 1987. "Ecomomic Evaluations of Unpaid Household Work: Africa, Asia, Latin America, and Oceania." *Women, Work, and Development Paper* # 14. Geneva: ILO.

———. 1984. "The Economic Value of Household Production: Methodological Problems." A Working Paper Presented at the Workshop on Conceptualizing the Household: Issues of Theory, Method, and Application. Cambridge, MA: Harvard Institute of Development.

———. 1983. "Does Housework Pay? A Product-Related Micreconomic Approach." *Journal of Women in Culture and Society* 9(1):108-119.

———. 1982. "Unpaid Work in the Household: A Review of Economic Evaluation Methods." *Women, Work, and Development Series* No. 1. Geneva: ILO.

Government of Zimbabwe. 1982. *Report of the Commission of Inquiry into the Agricultural Industry.* Harare: Government Printers.

———. 1986. *First Five Year National Development Plan 1980-1985.* Vol. 1. Harare: Government Printers.

Government of Zimbabwe Ministry of Health. 1985. *Mashonaland West Provincial Medical Director, Report on a Provincial Workshop on Health Services in Commercial Farming Areas.* Harare: mimeo.

Gray, Madi. 1980. "Race Ratios: the Politics of Population Control." In *Poverty and Population Control* edited by Lars Bondestam and Staffan Bergstrom. London: Academic Press.

Green, R. 1986a. *Sub-Saharan Africa: Poverty of Development, Development of Poverty*. Falmer, Sussex, UK: Institute of Development Studies Paper 218.

———. 1986b. *The IMF and Stabilisation in Sub-Saharan Africa: A Critical Review*. Falmer, Sussex, UK: Institute of Development Studies Paper 216.

Guillaume, A. 1988. *Santé de la reproduction en pays akyé*. Abidjan: ORSTOM, offset.

Guillaume, A. et S. Rey. 1988. "L'intérêt de l'approche anthropologique pour l'étude des comportements en matière de santé." Communication au Congrès Africain de Population, Dakar, Sénégal, 7-12 novembre.

Guillaume, A. et P. Vimard 1989. "Fostered and entrusted children." *Child environment and urbanization*. Documents and Reflexions 8:57-67. Abidjan: UNICEF West Central African Regional Office.

———. 1990. *Santé maternelle et infantile et dynamique familiale dans le Sud-Ouest de la Côte-d'Ivoire*. Abidjan: UNICEF, ENSEA, ORSTOM. (In press).

Guillaume, A. et A. Yapi Diahou. 1989. "Femmes, enfants et crise en Côte-d'Ivoire." Abidjan: Bureau Régional de l'UNICEF pour l'Afrique de l'Ouest.

Guyer, J. 1988. "Dynamic Approaches to Domestic Budgeting: Cases and Methods from Africa." In *Home Divided: Women and Income in the Third World*. Stanford: Stanford University Press.

———. 1986. "Intra-Household Processes and Farming Systems Research: Perspectives from Anthropology." In *Understanding Africa's Rural Households and Farming Systems*. Boulder: Westview Press.

———. 1980. "Household Budgets and Women's Income." African Studies Center, *Working Paper* #28. Boston: Boston University.

Hamilton, S., B. Popkin, and D. Spicer. 1984. *Women and Nutrition in Third World Countries*. New York: Bergin and Gravy Publishers, Inc.

Hanlon, Joseph. 1988. *NGO's and Other Aid Agencies in Mozambique*. European Conference Against South African Aggression in Mozambique and Angola, Bonn.

Hartmann, Betsy. 1987. *Reproductive Rights and Wrongs*. New York: Harper and Row.

Hermele, Kenneth. 1988. *Country Report, Mozambique*. Stockholm: Studies from the Research Division, the Planning Secretariat, SIDA.

Hofvander, Y., ed. 1983. *Maternal and Young Child Nutrition*. Excerpts from a United Nations Expert Group. Paris: UNESCO.

Hope, A. and S. Timmel. 1985. *Training for Transformation: A Handbook for Community Workers*. 3 vols. Gwere, Zimbabwe: Mambo Press.

Houyoux, J. et al. 1986. *Budgets Menagers à Kinshasa, Zaire*. Kinshasa: Département du Plan.

Howes, M. and R. Chambers. 1979. "Indigenous Technical Knowledge: Analysis, Implications, and Issues." *IDS Bulletin* 10(2):5-11.

ICRW. 1989. "Strengthening Women: Health Research Priorities for Women in Developing Countries." Washington, D.C.: International Center for Research on Women.

IITA. 1988. "Resource and Crop Management Program". *Annual Report 1988.* Ibadan, Nigeria: International Institute of Tropical Agriculture.

Imam, A. 1988. "Households and the Crisis in Africa." A paper presented at the Third General Assembly of the Association of African Women for Research and Development on The African Crisis and Women's Vision of the Way Out. Dakar: AAWORD.

INSEE. 1987. *Données Sociales, 1987.* Paris: Institut National de la Statistique et des Etudes Economiques.

———. 1990. *Données Sociales, 1990.* Paris: Institut National de la Statistique et des Etudes Economiques.

Institute of Race Relations. 1959. *Race Relations Survey, 1957- 1958.* Johannesburg: South African Institute of Race Relations.

Jiggins, J. 1989. "How Poor Women Earn Income in Sub-Saharan Africa and What Works Against Them." *World Development* 17(7):953-963.

Joekes, S. 1987. "Women's Work and Social Support for Child Care in the Third World." Washington, D.C.: ICRW.

Jones, C. W. 1986. "Intra-Household Bargaining in Response to the Introduction of New Crops: A Case Study from North Cameroon." In *Understanding Africa's Rural Households and Farming Systems,* edited by J. L. Moock. Boulder: Westview Press.

Jones, D. 1986. *Tea and Justice: British Tea Companies and Tea Workers of Bangladesh.* London: Bangladesh International Action Group.

Jordan, Phyllis. 1984. "Black Womanhood and National Liberation." *Sechaba.* African National Congress of South Africa.

Kanji, Najmi. 1989. Charging for Drugs in Africa: UNICEF's Bamako Initiative. *Health Policy and Planning* (2) 4:110-120.

Kanse, Mathias S. 1989. "Le CNR et les Femmes: de la Difficulté de Libérer la 'Moitié du Ciel'." *Politique Africaine* 33:66-72.

Kaufmann, G., R. Lesthaeghe, and D. Meekers. 1988. "Les caracteristiques et tendances du mariage." In *Population et Sociétés en Afrique au Sud du Sahara* sous la direction de Dominique Tabutin, 217-247. Paris: L'Harmattan.

Kazombaue, L. 1987. Interview with John Evenson, Lusaka. Unpublished.

Keita, Thérèse. 1983. "Niger: Le règne des apparences." In *Terre des Femmes* sous la direction d'Elisabeth Paquot, 102-108. Paris: La Découverte.

Kemp, C. 1986. "Unionisation: Do Basic Needs Matter?" Paper presented at the Workshop on People in Plantations: Means or Ends? Falmer, Sussex, UK: Institute of Development Studies.

Krug, Etienne. 1988. *Acessibilidade Economica aos Cuidados Fornecidos pelo Hospital Rural de Vilankulo*. (Economic Access to Care, Vilankulo Rural Hospital). Médecins Sans Frontières.

Kruks, Sonia and Ben Wisner. 1984. "The State, the Party and the Female Peasantry in Mozambique". *Journal of Southern African Studies* (1) 11:106-127.

Kuper, Leo. 1965. *An African Bourgeoisie: Race, Class, and Politics in South Africa*. New Haven and London: Yale University Press.

Lacoste-Dujardin, Camille. 1986. *Des Mères contres les Femmes: Maternité et Patriarchat au Maghreb*. Paris: Éditions La Découverte.

Ladjali, Malika. 1987. *L'espacement des Naissances en Algérie*. London: International Planned Parenthood Federation.

Ladjali, Malika and Claudine Chaulet. 1985. "Offre et Demande de Contraception: Reflexion sur l'Expérience Algérienne des Centres d'Espacement des Naissances." First Maghreb Congress on Family Planning, Tunis, October 1985.

Ladjali, Malika and Naheed Toubia. 1990. "Female Circumcision." *IPPF Medical Bulletin* 24(2):1-2.

Lallemand, S. 1980. "L'adoption des enfants chez les Kotokoli du Togo." *Anthropologie et sociétés*, 4(2):19-37.

Landman, Lynn. 1977. "Birth Control in India: The Carrot and the Road?" *Family Planning Perspectives* 9(3):101-110.

Leslie, J. 1987. "Women's Work and Child Nutrition in the Third World." Washington, D.C.: ICRW.

Leslie, Joanne, Margaret Lycette, and Myra Buvinic. 1986. *Weathering Economic Crises: the Crucial Role of Women in Health*. Washington: International Center for Research on Women.

Livingstone, D. 1857. *Missionary Travels and Researches in South Africa*. London: John Murray.

Locoh, Thérèse. 1984. *Fécondité et famille en Afrique de l'Ouest. Le Togo méridional contemporain*. Paris: INED, Travaux et documents, Cahier n° 107.

Loewenson, R. 1984. "The Health Status of Rural Labour Communities in Zimbabwe." MSc thesis, University of London.

———. 1985. "Evaluation of the Mashonaland West Farm Health Worker Scheme." Harare: Save The Children Fund (UK), mimeo.

———. 1986. "Farm Labour in Zimbabwe." *Health Policy and Planning* 1(1):48-57.

————. 1989. "The Health Implications of Changing Patterns of Large Scale Agricultural Production: the Zimbabwean Farmworker." Ph.D. thesis, University of London.

Loewenson, R. and A. Chinori. 1986. "The Socioeconomic Situation of Commercial Farmworkers in post Independence Zimbabwe." Harare: SIDA Report.

Loewenson, R., J. Zanza, and I. Mushayandebvu. "Interim Evaluation of the Bindura Farm Health Worker Project." Harare: Save The Children Fund (UK), mimeo.

Longe, O. G. 1985. "The Role of Women in Food Production, Processing, and Preservation." Paper presented at the seminar organized by the Institute of African Studies, University of Ibadan, Nigeria.

Longhurst, R. 1985. "Cropping Systems and Consumption: Cropping Systems and Household Food Security: Evidence from Three African Countries." *Food and Nutrition.* 11(2):10-16.

————. 1984. "The Energy Trap: Work, Nutrition and Child Malnutrition in Northern Nigeria." Cornell International Nutrition *Monograph Series* No. 13. Ithaca: Cornell University Program in International Nutrition.

————. 1982. "Resource Allocation and the Sexual Division of Labor: A Case Study of a Moslem Hausa Village in Northern Nigeria." In *Women and Development: The Sexual Division of Labor in Rural Societies,* edited by Lourdes Beneria, 97-117. New York: Praeger Scientific.

Longwe, S. H. 1985. "From Welfare to Empowerment: The Situation of Women in Development in Africa; A Post UN Women's Decade Update and Future Directions." A Paper presented to a NGO Africa Women's Task Force meeting, Nairobi, Kenya.

Lopes-Valcarcel, Beatriz Gonzalez, Miguel Sanchez Padron, J. Woodall, and E. Mello. 1988. "Study of the Economic Adjustment Policies on the Health Situation in Mozambique." World Health Organization, mimeo.

Loxley, John. 1988. "Economic Reform in Mozambique: Two Views. 1: Strategic Defeat or Tactical Retreat." *Southern Africa Report* (2) 4: 3-5.

Luckhardt, Ken and Brenda Wall. 1980. *Organise or Starve! The History of the South African Congress of Trade Unions.* New York: International Publishers.

Lunven, P. 1983. "The Value of Time-Use Data in Nutrition." *Food and Nutrition* 9(2):33-38.

MacGaffey, J. 1986. "Women and Class Formation in a Dependent Economy." In *Women and Class in Africa,* edited by C. Robertson and I. Berger, 161-177. New York: Africana.

———. 1988. "Evading Male Control: Women in the Second Economy in Zaire." In Stichter and Parpart, eds. 1988. *Patriarchy and Class*, 161-176. Boulder and London: Westview Press.

Mackintosh, Maureen. 1986. "Economic Policy Context and Adjustment Options in Mozambique". *Development and Change* 17:557- 81.

Machel, Samora. 1973. "Speech to the Conference of Organizaçao da Mulher Moçambicana." Maputo: mimeo.

Marks, Shula. 1988. "Class, Race and Gender in the South African Nursing Profession." Paper presented to the Canadian Association of African Studies, Queen's University, Kingston, Ontario, May 1988.

Marshall, G. A. 1965. "Women, Trade, and the Yoruba Family." Ph.D. Thesis. New York: Columbia University.

Marshall, Judith. 1988. "Why Shoot the Teacher? War and Education in Mozambique." African Studies Association Conference, Chicago.

———. 1989. *Structural Adjustment in Mozambique—the Human Dimension*. Ottawa: Canadian International Development Agency.

McSweeney, B. G. 1979. "Collection and Analysis of Data on Rural Women's Time Use." *Studies in Family Planning* 10(11/12):379-384.

Mebrahtu, S. 1989. "Women's Organizations in Nigeria: A Series of Case Studies." A paper prepared for the 1989 Laurie New Jersey Chair Seminar on Feminist Perspectives on Leadership, Power, and Diversity. New Brunswick: Rutgers University.

Mendelievich, E. 1980. *Le Travail des Enfants*. Geneva: International Labour Office.

Mernissi, F. 1983. *Sexe Idéologie Islam*. Paris: Editions Tierce.

Minces, J. 1990. *La Femme Voilée: L'Islam au Féminin*. Paris: Calmann-Lévy.

Ministère de la Santé. 1984. *Etats généraux de la Santé. La Santé en Côte-d'Ivoire, Situation actuelle et perspectives d'avenir*. Yamoussoukro: offset.

Mivumbi, N. 1988. "Le Marketing Social comme un des Moyens de Lutte contre le SIDA." Paper presented at N'sele Condom Conference, Kinshasa.

Monimart, Marie. 1989. *Femmes au Sahel*. Paris: Editions Karthala et OCDE/Club du Sahel.

Munslow, Barry. 1988. *Workshop on Economic Adjustment Programmes, the IMF and the World Bank*. European Conference Against South African Aggression in Mozambique and Angola, Bonn.

Mueller, E. 1979. "Time Use in Rural Botswana." A Paper Presented at a Seminar on the Rural Income Distribution Survey in Gabarone, Botswana. Ann Arbor: University of Michigan, Population Studies Center.

Naamane-Guessous, Soumaya. 1988. *Au-delà de Toute Pudeur*. Casablanca, Morocco: EDDIF.

Newbury, C. and B.G. Schoepf. 1989. "State, Peasantry and Agrarian Crisis in Zaire: Does Gender Make a Difference?" In *Women and the State in Africa*, edited by Jane L. Parpart and Kathleen A. Staudt, 91-110. Boulder, CO: Lynne Reinner.

N'Galy, B., R. W. Ryder, and K. Bila. 1988. "Human Immunodeficiency Virus Infection Among Employees at an African Hospital." *New England Journal of Medicine* 319(17):1123-1127.

N'Galy, B., R.W. Ryder and T.C. Quinn. 1989. Letter. *New England Journal of Medicine* 320 (24):1625.

Nieves, I. 1981. "A Balancing Act: Strategies to Cope With Work and Motherhood in Developing Countries." Paper prepared for the Roundtable on the Interface Between Poor Women's Nurturing Roles and Productive Responsibilities, Washington, D.C.: ICRW.

Noble, K.B. 1989. "Zaire's Battered Economy Inspires Optimism." *New York Times*, December 14: A6.

Nomvete, N. 1984. "The Participation of the Female Working Class in Trade Unions and in Labour Struggles in South Africa from 1950." Edinburgh: Edinburgh University Centre of African Studies *Occasional Papers* No. 6.

Nursing News. 1978. "The Nursing Bill: What It Means To Nurses" (Leader Article) 1:1.

Nursing News. 1983. "Warning Against Pitfalls of a Trade Union." (Leader Article) 7:1.

Nweke, F. I. and F. E. Winch. 1980. "Bases for Farm Resource Allocation in the Smallholder Cropping Systems of South Eastern Nigeria: A Case Study of Awka and Abakaliki Villages." *Discussion Paper* No. 4/80. Ibadan: Agricultural Economics, IITA.

OIT. 1985. *L'emploi des femmes en Afrique*. Rapport de synthèse dans six pays francophones (Bénin, Cameroun, Côte d'Ivoire, Madagascar, Sénégal, et Togo). Addis Abeba: Organisation Internationale du Travail, Programmes des Emplois et des Compétences Techniques pour l'Afrique.

Okeyo, A. P. 1979. "Women in Household Economy: Managing Multiple Roles." *Studies in Family Planning* 10(11/12):337-343.

Olayowe, J. E. 1985. "Factors Affecting the Role of Rural Women in Agricultural Production: A Survey of Rural Women in Oyo State, Nigeria." Paper presented at the seminar on Nigerian Women and National Development Organized by the Institute of African Studies. Ibadan: University of Ibadan.

OMS. 1971. "Planification familiale et les services de santé." Rapport d'un Comité d'experts de l'OMS. *Série de Rapports techniques* No. 476.

———. 1980. *Sixième Rapport sur la Situation Sanitaire dans le Monde, 1973-1977*. Partie II: Exposés par pays et territoires. Genève: Organisation Mondiale de la Santé.

Orford, H. J. L. 1976. "Letter." *South African Journal of Medicine.* February.

Oudin, X. 1984. "Population et emploi en Côte-d'Ivoire." Séminaire AISE/INSEE/MAROC sur les statistiques de l'emploi et du secteur non structuré, Rabat, octobre.

Parpart, J. L. 1988. "Sexuality and Power on the Zambian Copperbelt: 1926-1964." In *Patriarchy and Class*, edited by S. B. Stichter and J. L. Parpart, 115-138. Boulder: Westview Press

Paquot, E. 1983. "Excision et infibulation, pourquoi mutiler le sexe des petites filles?" In *Terre des Femmes* sous la direction d'Elisabeth Paquot, 338-340. Paris: La Découverte.

Perregaux, Christiane. 1990. *Femmes Sahraouies, Femmes du Désert*. Paris: L'Harmattan.

Pizurki, H., A. Mejia, I. Butter, and L. Ewart. 1987. *Women as Providers of Health Care*. Geneva: World Health Organization.

Ramji, Shiraz. 1987. *Growing Old in Mozambique Under Fire. A Study of Displaced Mozambican Elderly Living in Mozambique and Zimbabwe*. Help the Aged.

Republic of South Africa. 1946. *Medicine, Dentistry and Pharmacy Nursing Act No. 45 of 1944 as amended by Nursing Act 12 of 1946*. Part III, Section 12(2):157.

République Française. 1981. *Gabon: Analyse et Conjonctures*. Ministère de la Coopération et du Développement. Mimeo.

République Gabonaise. 1980. *Annuaire Statistique du Gabon, 1976- 1980*. Ministère de la Planification et de l'Aménagement du Territoire, Direction Générale de la Statistique et des Etudes Economiques.

Riddell, R. 1979. "Zimbabwe: Problems for the Economy." *ODI Review* 1:24-36.

———. 1981. *Report of the Commission of Inquiry into Incomes, Prices and Conditions of Service*. Harare: Government

Roberts, Penelope. 1988. "Rural Women's Access to Labor in West Africa." In *Patriarchy and Class: African Women in the Home and the Workforce*, edited by Sharon B. Stichter and Jane L. Parpart, 97-114. Boulder and London: Westview Press.

Rogers, B. L. 1983. "The Internal Dynamics of Households: A Critical Factor in Development." A Paper Prepared for the Agency for International Development Nutrition and Development Project. Paper No. 83-2. Washington, D.C.: Government Printing Office.

Roux, Edward. 1972. *Time Longer Than Rope*. Madison and London: The University of Wisconsin Press.

Rukarangira wa Nkera and B. G. Schoepf. 1989. "Réactions de la Société Zaïroise envers le SIDA." Paper presented at the V International Conference on AIDS, Montreal, 5 June 1989. Abstract No. 7134.

Sabo, Lois E. and Joachim S. Kibirige. 1989."Political Violence and Eritrean Health Care." *Social Science and Medicine* 28(7):677- 684.

Salvage, J. 1985. *The Politics of Nursing.* London: Heinemann.

Savané, Marie-Angélique. 1983. "Sénégal: Les carcans de la tradition." In *Terre des Femmes* sous la direction d'Elisabeth Paquot, 114-116. Paris: La Découverte.

Schoepf, B. G. 1981. "Women in the Informal Economy of Lubumbashi." Paper presented at the annual meeting of the African Studies Association, Bloomington, Indiana, mimeo.

———. 1988. "Sex, Blood and Condoms: 'Traditional' Healers and Community-Based AIDS Prevention in Zaire." Paper presented at the 88th Annual Meeting of American Anthropological Association.

Schoepf, B. G. and C. Schoepf. 1981. "Zaire's Rural Development: Problems and Prospects." In *The Role of US Universities in Rural and Agricultural Development,* edited by B. G. Schoepf, 243-257. Tuskegee, Ala: Tuskegee Institute.

———. 1988. "Zaire's Rural Development: Problems and Prospects." In *The Heterosexual Transmission of AIDS in Africa,* edited by D. Koch-Weser and H. Vanderschmidt, 265- 280. Boston: Abt.

Schoepf, B. G. et al. 1988a. "AIDS and Society in Central Africa: A View from Zaire." In *AIDS in Africa: Social and Policy Impact,* edited by N. Miller and R. Rockwell, 211-235. Lewiston, N.Y.: Edwin Mellen.

———. 1988b. "AIDS, Women and Society in Central Africa." In *AIDS 1988: AAAS Symposium Papers,* edited by R. Kulstad, 175- 181. Washington, D.C.: AAAS.

Searle, Charlotte. 1965. *The History of the Development of Nursing in South Africa 1952-1960.* Cape Town: Struik.

Secçâo de Nutriçâo. 1989. *Sumario da Situaçâo Nutricional em Moçambique no ano 1988.* (Summary of the Nutritional Situation in Mozambique in 1988). Maputo: Direcçâo Nacional de Saude.

Shor, P. and P. Freire. 1978. *Pedagogy in Process.* New York: Seabury.

Sircar, K., J. Sajhau, A. Mavamukundau, and R. Sukanja. 1985. "The Socio-Economic Implications of Structural Changes in Plantations in Asian Countries." ILO Working Paper SAP 2.1/WP2, Geneva: International Labour Office.

Slesinger, D., B. Christenson, and E. Caukley. 1986. "Health and Mortality of Migrant Farm Children." *Social Science and Medicine* 23(1):65-74.

Sobukhwe, Robert. 1949. *Speeches of Mangaliso Sobukhwe from 1949-1959 and Documents of the Pan Africanist Congress Azania.* New

York: PAC of Azania, Office of the Chief Representative to the United States and the Caribbean.

South African Nursing Association. 1988. "Proposed Amendments to the Constitution of the South African Nursing Association." Circular No. 12, mimeo.

Spiro, H. M. 1980a. "The Domestic Economy and Rural Time Budgets." *Agricultural Economics Discussion Paper* No. 6/80. Ibadan: IITA.

———. 1980b. "The Role of Women Farming in Oyo State, Nigeria: A Case Study in Two Rural Communities." *Agricultural Economics Discussion Paper* No. 7/8. Ibadan: IITA.

———. 1985. *Women's Roles and Gender Differences in Development: The Ilora Farm Settlement in Nigeria*. West Hartford: Kumarian Press.

Standing, Guy. 1989. "Global Feminization through Flexible Labor." *World Development* 17(7):1077-1095.

Steiner, K. G. 1984. "Intercropping in Tropical Smallholder Agriculture with Special Reference to West Africa." GTZ, Eschborn, Germany.

Stern, E. M. 1982. "Collective Bargaining: Means of Conflict Resolution." *Nursing Administration Quarterly* 6:9-12.

Stichter, S. B. and J. L. Parpart. 1988. "Introduction: Towards a Materialist Perspective on African Women." In *Patriarchy and Class: African Women in the Home and the Workforce*, edited by S. B. Stichter and J. L. Parpart, 1-26. Boulder and London: Westview Press.

Stoneman, C. 1981. *Zimbabwe's Inheritance*. London: Macmillan.

Strauss, S. A. 1981. *Legal Handbook for Nurses and Health Personnel*. Cape Town: King Edward Trust.

Sudarkasa, N. 1975. "Where Women Work: A Study of Yoruba Women in the Marketplace and in the Home." *Anthropological Paper* No. 53. Ann Arbor: University of Michigan Museum of Anthropology.

Summerfield, Derek. 1988. "A New Kind of Child Abuse". *Lancet* i:8590.

Tarrab, Gilbert. 1989. *Femmes et Pouvoirs au Burkina Faso*. Paris: L'Harmattan.

Turshen, Meredeth. 1984. *The Political Ecology of Disease in Tanzania*. New Brunswick, NJ: Rutgers University Press.

———. 1986. "Workers Health in Africa." *Review of African Political Economy* 36:25-29.

———. 1989. *The Politics of Public Health*. New Brunswick, NJ: Rutgers University Press.

UN. 1987. "Measuring and Valuing Women's Participation in the Informal Sector of the Economy." A Report of the Statistical Office, *UN Secretariat Working Paper* No. 6. New York: UN.

UNICEF. 1989. *Children on the Frontline. The Impact of Apartheid, Destabilization and Warfare on Children in Southern and South Africa*. New York: UNICEF.

———. 1989. *Femmes et Enfants au Mali: Une analyse de situation.* Paris: L'Harmattan.

UNICEF, WHO, and the World Bank. 1987. *La Contribution de la Plannification Familiale à L'amélioration de la Santé des Femmes et des Enfants.* Report of a conference held in Nairobi, Kenya.

Urdang, Stephanie. 1989. *And Still They Dance. Women, War, and the Struggle for Change in Mozambique.* New York: Monthly Review Press.

Van Hoffen, M. ed. 1986. *Commercial Agriculture in Zimbabwe, 1985/1986.* Harare: Modern Farming Publications.

Vidal, C. et M. Le Pape. 1986. *Pratiques de Crise et Conditions Sociales à Abidjan 1979-1985.* Abidjan: Centre ORSTOM de Petit-Bassam.

Vock, Jane. 1988. "Demographic Theories and Women's Reproductive Labor." In *Patriarchy and Class: African Women in the Home and Workforce,* edited by S. B. Stichter and J. L. Parpart, 81-96. Boulder and London: Westview Press.

Wagatsuma, Takashi. 1971. "The Abortion Program in Japan." *Journal of Reproductive Medicine* 7(1):30-33.

Walt, Gillian and Angela Melamed (eds.) 1984. *Mozambique: Towards a People's Health Service.* London: Zed Press.

Walu Engundu. 1987. "Budgets Ménagers des Femmes à Kinshasa." Report to the World Bank, Washington, D.C. June.

Weiner, D., S. Moyo, B. Munslow, and P. O'Keefe. 1985. "Land Use and Agricultural Productivity in Zimbabwe." *Journal of Modern African Studies* 23(2):251-285.

White, B. 1984. "Measuring Time Allocation, Decision Making and Agrarian Changes Affecting Rural Women: Examples from Recent Research in Indonesia." *IDS Bulletin* 15(1):18-32.

WHO. 1989. *Coverage of Maternity Care: A Tabulation of Available Information.* Geneva: WHO Division of Family Health, second edition.

Whyte, B. 1957. *Nursing Times* July 12, 786.

Williams, Frieda. 1982. "Interview." *Women's Committee Newsletter of the Anti-Apartheid Movement,* 5.

World Bank. 1983. *Zimbabwe: Population, Health and Nutrition.* Washington, D.C.: World Bank.

———. 1986. *World Development Report.* Washington, D.C.

———. 1988. World Development Report. Washington, D.C.

Wright, Marcia. 1985. *Health Activism in Southern Africa: Nurse and Primary Health Care.* Proceedings of the First Workshop of the Project, 'Poverty, Health and the State in Southern Africa,' November. New York: Columbia University.

Wuyts, Mark. 1989. *Economic Management and Adjustment Policies in Mozambique.* Conference on Economic Crisis and Third World Countries: Impact and Response, Institute of Social and Economic Research, University of the West Indies, and United Nations Research Institute for Social Development, Kingston.

Zimbabwe Agricultural Workers Union. 1981. "A Brief Address to the Fiet Southern Africa Advisory Council." Harare: ZAWU, mimeo.

Contributors

JULIE CLIFF is an Australian physician who has worked in Mozambique since 1976, first in the Central Hospital, Maputo, and then in the preventive services in the Ministry of Health. She has documented the impact of South African destabilization on health in Mozambique (*Social Science and Medicine*) and more specifically on maternal and child health (*Journal of Tropical Pediatrics*). She recently had a year's leave as an international fellow in epidemiology at the U.S. Centers for Disease Control.

AGNÈS GUILLAUME is a demographer with ORSTOM, the French Scientific Research Institute for Cooperative Development. She spent three years in Côte d'Ivoire carrying out research on reproductive health.

QUARRAISHA KHAN is a microbiologist from South Africa who recently received a master's degree from Columbia University.

MALIKA LADJALI is an Algerian physician who directs her country's maternal and child health and family planning program. She is currently on a two-year leave of absence with the International Planned Parenthood Federation in London.

JENNY LINDSAY holds a Ph.D. in Politics from Leeds University, where she also obtained the M.A. and B.A. degrees. She teaches sociology and politics at the Open University. Currently she is involved in an electoral study in Namibia, together with members of the Leeds Politics Department.

RENÉ LOEWENSON is a Zimbabwean currently lecturing in community medicine in the University of Zimbabwe Medical School. Since independence in 1980 she has carried out research on plantations, assessing socioeconomic and health status, the impact of Ministry of Health primary health care programs, and the impact of occupational hazards such as pesticide use. She has also been involved in training in these areas with the agricultural workers union (GAPWUZ).

NONCEBA LUBANGA received her nursing training in South Africa and England. Since coming to the United States in 1970, she has obtained a Master's Degree in Public Health from Columbia University. She is on the faculty of the Community Health Nursing Division at the Columbia University School of Nursing. She is also a health services coordinator at Talbot Perkins Children's Services in New York City. She is active in the Committee on Health in South Africa and other support groups.

SABA MEBRAHTU is an Ethiopian sociologist who completed two years of doctoral fieldwork in Nigeria, funded by the Ford Foundation through the International Institute of Tropical Agriculture, Nigeria, and the Dietary Management of Diarrhea Program of the Johns Hopkins University. She is currently at Cornell University, Population and Development Program, completing her dissertation.

PAYANZO NTSOMO is a Zairian sociologist who obtained his Ph.D. from Northwestern University in 1974. A specialist in urban sociology and education, he has worked as a development consultant and in the administration of Zairian higher education. He currently teaches at the Institut National de Pédagogie and the University of Kinshasa. He also represented the district in which the CONNAISSIDA project took place in the National Legislative Council.

RUKARANGIRA WA NKERA, a Zairian physician and public health specialist, is codirector of Project CONNAISSIDA and a public health specialist with experience in medical and economic anthropology. He is currently a Takemi Fellow in International Health at the Harvard School of Public Health. He serves as a consultant to the World Health Organization's Global Program on AIDS.

BROOKE GRUNDFEST SCHOEPF, a medical and economic anthropologist and professional human relations trainer, directs Project CONNAISSIDA. She has taught and researched development issues in Africa since 1974, when she joined the Rockefeller Foundation's field staff at the Université Nationale du Zaire in Lubumbashi. She currently is an Evelyn Green Davis Fellow at the Bunting Institute, Radcliffe College, and is writing a book, *Sex, Gender and Society: The Sociocultural Production of AIDS in Zaire.*

CLAUDE SCHOEPF is an agricultural economist with five years of field research and consulting experience in Zaire. He provides administrative backup and data analysis for CONNAISSIDA.

MEREDETH TURSHEN holds a doctorate in politics and teaches at the Rutgers University Faculty of Planning and at the University of Medicine and Dentistry of New Jersey—Robert Wood Johnson Medical School. She worked for twelve years in the United Nations system with UNICEF and WHO. She has published two books, *The Political Ecology of Disease in Tanzania* (1984) and *The Politics of Public Health* (1989).

WALU ENGUNDU, who obtained a *licence* in economic anthropology in 1977, is a Zairian research associate at the Centre de Recherche en Sciences Humaines in Kinshasa. She has conducted field research on health and development issues and is preparing a doctoral thesis on "Women's Survival Strategies in Kinshasa in the Face of Economic Crisis."

Index